THE SCIENCE OF
BRAIN HEALTH

The Simple 7 Step Solution to Prevent the Nightmare of Alzheimer's

Dr. John Zielonka

Health and Wellness Canada

Ottawa, ON Canada

www.drjohnzielonka.com

The Science of Brain Health

The Simple 7 Step Solution to Prevent

the Nightmare of Alzheimer's

by Dr. John Zielonka

Copyright © 2020 Dr. John Zielonka

ALL RIGHTS RESERVED

First Printing – May 2020

ISBN: 978-1-09582-318-7

The information in this book is for educational purposes only. It is not intended as medical advice nor to diagnose, treat or cure any disease. Dr. Zielonka encourages you to make your own health care decisions based upon your research and in partnership with a qualified health care professional. The taking of prescription drugs and vitamin supplements can have both beneficial and adverse effects on your health. All readers are strongly advised to personally consult a qualified health care professional for conditions specific to their own health and not to rely solely on the information in this book.

NO PART OF THIS BOOK MAY BE REPRODUCED IN ANY FORM, BY PHOTOCOPYING OR BY ANY ELECTRONIC OR MECHANICAL MEANS, INCLUDING INFORMATION STORAGE OR RETRIEVAL SYSTEMS, WITHOUT PERMISSION IN WRITING FROM THE COPYRIGHT OWNER/AUTHOR

Printed in the U.S.A.

0 1 2 3 4 5

DEDICATION

This book is dedicated to all of those who have witnessed or experienced the nightmare of Alzheimer's and who wishes to help prevent this dreaded disease from ever occurring in the first place.

ACKNOWLEDGEMENTS

A special thank-you to my always appreciated proof-reader Carmen Danner and to Ryan Biore (ryanurz) from 99designs for his wonderful book cover design.

TABLE OF CONTENTS

Part One – Introduction 13

1. My Goal for You 15
2. Flip a Coin 17
3. The Nightmare of Alzheimer's - The Basics 19

Part Two – Understanding Health and Science ... 23

4. Understanding Health and How it Applies to Alzheimer's 25
5. The Health Continuum 33
6. Society's Paradigms of Health 39
7. Why Science isn't so Scientific 45
8. Brain Health and Prescription Drugs – Why this Approach won't Work 53
9. The 3 Biggest Reasons Society has it Wrong – The 17-Year Problem 61
10. Dr. Z's 12 Big Ideas You Need to Understand 65

Part Three – Your Brain and Alzheimer's 71

11. How the Brain Works: Neurons, Neuroplasticity and

Neurotransmitters.. 73

12. Alzheimer's – Is the Nightmare Inevitable?............................ 81

13. The 3 Theories of Alzheimer's… and Why they're Wrong...... 87

14. Which Means the Testing is Wrong as Well......................... 91

15. The Six Types of Alzheimer's 95

16. The Role of Genetics.. 99

17. Type 3 Diabetes 103

18. Chronic Brain Inflammation 107

19. Toxins 111

20. Trauma 117

Part Four – The Simple 7 Step Solution 121

21. The Simple 7 Step Solution – The Overview...................... 123

22. Proper Diagnosis.. 129

23. Apple Juice and Stewed Mosquitoes 133

24. The Healthy Brain Diet 137

25. Fasting and Brain Health 141

26. Do I Really Need To Take Vitamins? The Question Answered Once and For All 145

27. Biochemistry 101 – The Role of Vitamins in Preventing Alzheimer's 155

28. Where Do I Buy My Vitamin Supplements?............................ 171

29. Brain Detoxification and True Cellular Detox........................ 177

30. Gut Biome 185

31. The 5 Keys to Health 187

32. Your Thoughts 195

Part Five – After the Fact 199

33. What Do You Do Now?.. 201

34. The Only Logical Choice.. 205

35. Additional Help 207

36. Dr. John Zielonka 209

"A masterful blend of both the latest science-based evidence combined with a practical, common-sense, simple step-by-step formula to prevent the nightmare from ever happening in the first place. Having witnessed what Dr. John Zielonka calls the nightmare of Alzheimer's far too many times to count, this book is long overdue".

Dr. Alan Weinstein, Functional Neurologist

"This book is a must-read for those wishing to prevent Alzheimer's as well as for those who are carrying the tremendous burden of caring for those who currently suffer from it. Congratulations to Dr. Zielonka for exposing the false dogma around this disease and providing a practical solution that everyone can achieve".

Dr. David Zamikoff, Natural Healing Arts Medical Ctr

ADDITIONAL RESOURCES FROM DR. ZIELONKA

Complimentary:

1. Please visit www.DrJohnZielonka.com to watch Dr. Zielonka's masterclass discussing his Signature Coaching Program – "The Simple 7 Step Solution to Prevent the Nightmare of Alzheimer's".

2. Please visit www.DrJohnZielonka.com to listen to Dr. Zielonka's internet radio interview discussing "The 5 Keys to Health".

3. For those wishing to learn cutting edge information on multiple aspects of health, readers are encouraged to subscribe to Dr. Zielonka's leading health podcast "The Science of Brain Health" available on iTunes and at www.DrJohnZielonka.com.

4. To learn more about true brain detoxification please visit www.DrJohnZielonka.com.

PREAMBLE
NEWSFLASH

As this book is going to print, events are occurring in the news that have spurred me to write this "newsflash" to add to the beginning of my book.

I remember some five years ago when I was being interviewed on a US Internet Radio station. I was discussing how unfortunate it was that for many, old age simply brought more pain and suffering. I referenced a television commercial at the time put out by the Heart and Stroke Association that stated that the average Canadian would spend the last ten years of their life in pain and suffering. The interviewer responded "the last ten – here in the US it's the last twenty".

How sad is that? You're born, you grow up, and you spend your entire life working hard to provide for your family only to spend the last ten to twenty years in pain and suffering. With Alzheimer's, it's even worse. Not only are you dealing with this pain and suffering, you eventually get to the point where you've forgotten your family that you love and whom you provided for your entire life.

It was this realization that prompted me to write this book.

Even with everything that I have been teaching my patients about health over the past 28 years, whether it was how to prevent heart disease, cancer, diabetes or optimize health, Alzheimer's and its seemingly inevitable nightmare was on the rise. It just didn't make sense to spend an entire lifetime's worth of effort to prevent heart disease and cancer only to end up with Alzheimer's.

At the time of this book's first printing there are four current and relevant news stories;

1. Canada has announced that it is developing a new directive to deal with Alzheimer's to be released later this year,
2. A new vaccine for Alzheimer's is undergoing trials,
3. Canada has a new food guide.
4. Dr. Oz is talking about a new blood test for Alzheimer's.

But as you will discover in this book, none of these approaches will do anything to successfully cure or prevent Alzheimer's. This is not pessimism, rather, I consider myself an optimistic realist. These approaches will not work because it's simply more of the same. That's what this book is for – a different step-by-step solution that works.

I have this saying in my office. "Hope is nice, but action is better". The science is clear and you need to act. You can no longer wait for the government to save you or for the latest miracle cure that is never coming. You need to take action today if you are to prevent this nightmare of a disease from ever happening in the first place. You'll find the answers on exactly how to do that and much more right here in this book.

PART ONE
INTRODUCTION

CHAPTER 1
MY GOAL FOR YOU

If you've ever been one of the thousands of people that I have been privileged to help in my health centre over the past quarter century, you would discover that one of the main tenets of my care is "Health By Choice – Not By Chance". As such, you get to choose what your goal is after reading this book. My goal, on the other hand, in both writing it, and you reading it, is twofold;

1. **Awareness and Knowledge**

    Alzheimer's is a dreaded disease. In fact, you will see me refer to it as a *nightmare* many times throughout these chapters. My first goal in writing this book was to make you aware that, contrary to many people's beliefs, **it is preventable in 90% of cases based on the science** and in some cases in the early stages even reversible. Furthermore, my desire is to share with you the knowledge of exactly how to do this.

2. **Take Action**

    You can have all the knowledge in the world but if I don't

convince you to take action, then we've accomplished nothing. And to be blunt, why should I have to *convince* you to prevent Alzheimer's? Shouldn't it be a given that you would want to?

The truth is that contained within this book is **the solution** - a logical, real, science-based solution that exists today to prevent a nightmare that you are likely to experience. The only problem is that the vast majority, including most doctors, have no idea that such a solution even exists. As such, it may be 10 or 20 years before you accept this fact and by then it may be too late.

Please, for the sake of you and your family, read, share and take action on the seven steps necessary to prevent Alzheimer's and other forms of dementia from ever happening in the first place. Your livelihood and that of your loved ones depends upon it.

Dr. Zielonka's Health Thought:

**Hope is nice...
but action is better**

CHAPTER 2
FLIP A COIN

Let's make this as straightforward as possible. Please pull out a coin and flip it. But just before you flip it imagine that instead of heads and tails the two sides of this coin are cancer and heart disease. That's right, instead of heads and tails the average person will flip heads – you'll die of heart disease or tails – you'll die of cancer.

"But wait," you say. "With all the latest advances in technology and drugs, aren't people living longer and longer and aren't we preventing disease?" Actually, no we're not. The idea that cancer patients are living longer is a myth due mostly to earlier detection and how survival rates are calculated but that's for another book or my podcast. And if you're waiting for the miracle cure or latest vaccine, good luck with that. The truth is that millions continue to die and suffer with disease that is mostly preventable.

"But wait again," you say. "I'm smart enough to make wise health choices consistently throughout my life to prevent cancer and heart disease." Great – then flip that coin again. Chances are you'll live past 85 years of age. Once you hit 85, you have that same 50-50 chance that you'll suffer from Alzheimer's or some other form of dementia. And if you have a spouse, either you'll have it or you'll be taking care of your spouse who does. Do you really want to leave your health and your life to the flip of a coin? More so, do you want to spend a lifetime ensuring that you don't get cancer or heart disease only to come back to that same coin again? By following my Simple 7 Step program in this book, you will discover that all of this is preventable from ever happening in the first place.

Health Fact #1:

If you plan to live to 85 years of age and beyond, you have a 1 in 2 chance that you will suffer from Alzheimer's or some other form of dementia.

CHAPTER 3

THE NIGHTMARE OF ALZHEIMER'S - THE BASICS

Alzheimer's is a progressive neurological disease affecting memory and thought. It leaves its victims with significant loss of memory to the point where they fail to recognize their closest friends and loved ones and forget how to perform everyday tasks. It can result in severe mental confusion and anxiety as well as extreme loneliness. It is a terrible way to spend the last years of your life for both the person afflicted and those who care for them.

You die before you die

In reality, Alzheimer's is such a dreaded disease that you die before you die. Your memories, life experiences and remembering how to do the most basic of activities are all gone.

Rose's Story

I have been the primary caregiver for my mother with Alzheimer's for the past 10 years. She is 74 and seems to get worse every day little by little yet she seems strong enough otherwise that she may still live on for years. It is unbelievably cruel to see someone you love so much waste away mentally by this terrible disease day by day by day.

I can't begin to put into words how devastating this is for her and for me. She is the one suffering but so am I. Not only is this a terrible way for anyone to spend the last 10 or 20 years of their life but it has handcuffed me 24/7 both mentally and physically. I know it may sound selfish to some but I'm only 57. Since age 47 my life has drastically changed and there is no end in sight. I have no one else and the thought that I (and she) have been condemned to spend the rest of our lives like this goes way beyond unfair.

We've been given a lifetime sentence for a crime we never committed. There is no retirement in sight or any plans for the future. I have accepted giving up my life for my mother but the worst part is that the end result is inevitable. My biggest fear, however; is that I will get Alzheimer's before my mother passes away. I'm only 7 years away from when she got it. How will I ever take care of her then and who will take care of me?

Alzheimer's disease is currently the 6th leading cause of death in the United States affecting over 5.7 million Americans and over 50 million worldwide. What's worse is that if you plan on living to 85, nearly half of the population (47%) will be affected. Even worse, it is really the only cause of death among the top 10 in the United States (yes – people do die as a result of Alzheimer's) where **medical treatments are unable to cure, prevent or slow the progression of the disease to any appreciable degree.**

Health Fact #2:

There is currently no drug or medical treatment of any kind that is able to cure, prevent or slow the progression of Alzheimer's to any appreciable degree.

PART TWO

UNDERSTANDING HEALTH AND SCIENCE

CHAPTER 4

UNDERSTANDING HEALTH AND HOW IT APPLIES TO ALZHEIMER'S

If you're at all familiar with any of my work, you probably won't be surprised that this book is about more than just Alzheimer's. Why? Because it's necessary if we are to truly understand Alzheimer's.

Let's take a step back because if we're going to prevent Alzheimer's we need to take a different approach. Obviously the current approach simply isn't working and never will. In fact, let's step right back to the beginning and a concept sorely lacking in most aspects of our so called health-care system – let's discuss "health". If we don't truly understand health, we'll never understand Alzheimer's and other forms of dementia nor will we ever be able to prevent it.

You've heard your grandparents say it, and maybe even your parents: "Without your health, you have nothing." And yet, if that's true, why do we have so many unhealthy people in this world, especially those who have the means and ability to be better? If I were to ask you what the most important aspect of health was, you might say: "Well, it's nutrition, of course." After all, you are what you eat. Without the proper foods how can one ever expect to maximize their health?

Others would say: "Well yes, nutrition is important, but exercise is the key to health." Your body was meant to move until the day you die. Keeping active improves blood flow, heart function and mental clarity and reduces stress. It improves strength, helps to prevent osteoporosis and reduces the effects of aging.

Others say: "It's my doctor. She's the one responsible for my health. Besides, with all the newest and latest drugs I'll live forever and soon I'll be able to have an *artificial everything*."

Others would say the exact opposite. "The last thing I want is a drug. It's the natural approach that's most important. Give me my chiropractor, massage therapist, naturopath and vitamins."

But what if I were to tell you that none of these is right? Most of them are extremely beneficial and in fact essential for true optimum health, but they're not the single most important factor. What if I were to tell you that the single most important factor in helping you achieve optimum health is **what you believe?** Now don't get me wrong – we're not going to wish Alzheimer's away – in fact, exactly the opposite, this book is based on the latest and best science. But, without a doubt, your current belief system may unknowingly be helping or harming you in your quest for optimum health and, more often than not, is leading you to an early grave. Your views on health, the action you take (or don't take), the effort you're prepared to make and your knowledge of health are only the beginning. Please understand that we have been engrained with a belief system and set of paradigms that is unique to each of us. And it is this belief system that results in the everyday choices we make that impact our health, whether positively or negatively.

These belief systems are engrained in us from birth by our parents, society, and "health-care" system and are perpetuated on a daily basis. For example, imagine two children, Mary and Johnny. Mary is like most children who spend more time in front of the TV than they probably should and as a result is exposed to marketing and advertising on a daily basis. How much so? Well, it is estimated that the average child from birth to age 18 will be exposed to 20,000 ads for drugs. That is the equivalent of getting a drug ad at every single meal Mary has from birth until she reaches adulthood. So at every single breakfast, lunch and dinner Mary has, she is essentially told: "If you have a pain, take a pill. If you feel sick, pop a pill. If you want to feel better, take a drug. Don't worry about the underlying cause, just mask the symptoms. You don't have to be responsible for your health because there will always be a pill. And it must be the right approach because the doctor said it was okay, my parents gave it to me and everyone else seems to be doing it."

Now imagine Johnny. Johnny's parents weren't overly zealous anti-drug parents (if there is such a thing) but rather they led by example. They made healthy choices for Johnny from birth. Drugs were rarely needed, if ever. Johnny learned that healthy food could also taste good and his family was always active. Imagine the different beliefs that Johnny and Mary would have and how this would impact their health for the rest of their lives.

Of course, this goes well beyond upbringing and well beyond the use of drugs. It also goes beyond education as you can have two qualified health professionals read the exact same scientific study and yet come to two completely different conclusions.

Now imagine if everyone had the *right* beliefs about health. What do I mean by *right* beliefs given that there is no such thing as a right or wrong belief? I mean imagine if everyone had beliefs that led to better health. After all, isn't it amazing to see how some will exert more effort to defend their right to a belief that will make them unhealthy than they will to be healthy? In essence, they are arguing that they have the right to be unhealthy. And whether your belief is right or wrong, it will have an impact on your health whether you believe it or not.

One of the biggest paradigms and beliefs necessary for optimum health is to properly define what the word "health" actually means. If you think you already know, you may be sadly mistaken. How else do you explain the needless pain, suffering and deaths from chronic degenerative conditions such as heart disease, cancer and Alzheimer's in countries that not only have the ability to be better but are supposed to know better?

What is Health?

After a quarter century of studying optimal health, after treating thousands of patients and educating thousands more in my workshops and lectures, I am convinced that the majority of the population does not even know what the word "health" means. (In fact, you could be one of them, no matter how healthy you think you are.) Who are the biggest culprits? Most politicians and most health professionals. And yet if this is true, how on earth can we ever achieve optimal health? How can we expect to have healthy beliefs if we don't even know what the word "health" means? If you think I'm exaggerating, I challenge you to take this simple test right now. Simply define the word "health". Please. Pause for just a moment and before flipping to the next page simply write out or say aloud your definition of the word health.

Please define "health"

So how did you do? If you said being pain-free or feeling great, then you're wrong. While you want to feel great and certainly don't want to be in pain, it has nothing to do with the definition of health. And yet, not only have I heard other health professionals define health as pain-free, but our entire health-care system makes this a priority. The actual dictionary definition of "health", from both Dorland's medical dictionary and the World Health Organization, is:

HEALTH

> "The OPTIMAL state of physical, mental and social well being - and not merely the absence of disease or infirmity."
>
> Dorland's Medical Dictionary
> 27th edition and the
> World Health Organization

Please appreciate that there are three key points to this definition. They are not just telling you what health is: they are actually telling you what health isn't. The fact that you do not have some disease or infirmity (or pain) does not mean that you are healthy. I am not aware of any other word in the English language that is defined in this way. It is like saying an apple is a fruit which is not a banana. Secondly, health is holistic: physical, mental and social well-being (I would include spiritual as well). And, last but not least, by its own definition it is the *optimal* state. So if you're not 100%, you're not really healthy. As such, I'm guilty of being redundant every time I use the phrase *optimum health* as by its own definition health is already optimal. That is why health could also be defined as 100% functioning of 100 % of your body, mind and spirit 100% of the time.

Now imagine if the whole world not only knew this but actually acted upon it.

Health – "100% function of 100% of your body, mind and spirit, 100% of the time"

This concept is extremely important in our solution for Alzheimer's because, as you will soon discover, most of society and our sick-care system is completely wrong about Alzheimer's and other forms of dementia; why we get it, and how to fix it.

CHAPTER 5

THE HEALTH CONTINUUM

Our health - and lack of it - can be plotted along the health continuum. At one end of the health continuum (the far left) is true optimal health. At the other end (the far right) is death. And yes, our physical bodies are all eventually leading to the far right unless you "believe" in quantum physics in which case your energy and atoms will go on forever. But what if I were to tell you that you have a significant say not only in where you are along the continuum but also in how quickly or slowly you move along it?

We all understand that disease begins long before any symptoms appear. This is true of heart disease where your arteries first begin clogging long before you experience any chest pain or shortness of breath. This is true of cancer where cells mutate long before any symptoms appear. This is even true in other health professions such as dentistry where the cavity begins long before you feel the toothache or in chiropractic where the vertebral subluxation (spinal misalignment resulting in nerve dysfunction) begins long before you feel the back pain or headache. And of course, this is certainly true in Alzheimer's and other forms of dementia where changes in the brain occur long before any symptoms are noticed.

Once **Symptoms Appear** (please refer to the chart on the next page), they are often ignored or masked and disease or sick care is not sought until the disease has progressed. This often progresses to **Serious Disease** and eventually **Death**. Where is our sick care system focused? Between disease care sought and **Serious Disease** hoping to prevent **Death**. To understand that this system will never work one only needs to look at demographics.

25 years ago, 1 in 10 people were aged 65+. 15 years from now it will be more than 1 in 5. If you practice optimal health, then being aged 65+ is not a problem. However, in today's society being aged 65+ means you are that much more likely to be between **Disease Care Sought** and **Serious Disease** or even **Serious Disease** and **Death**. If our government currently spends more money on health care than anything else just to achieve such a poor system, if there is no more money in sight, and if the number of people moving towards **Serious Disease** is just going to increase as the population gets older, then how can any rational person ever expect that our system can be fixed? Obviously we need a new approach, a new paradigm and a new belief, which is simply to focus on the exact opposite end of the health continuum.

Further appreciate that there is a significant difference between **Prevention** and **Early Detection**. **Prevention** (optimal nutrition,

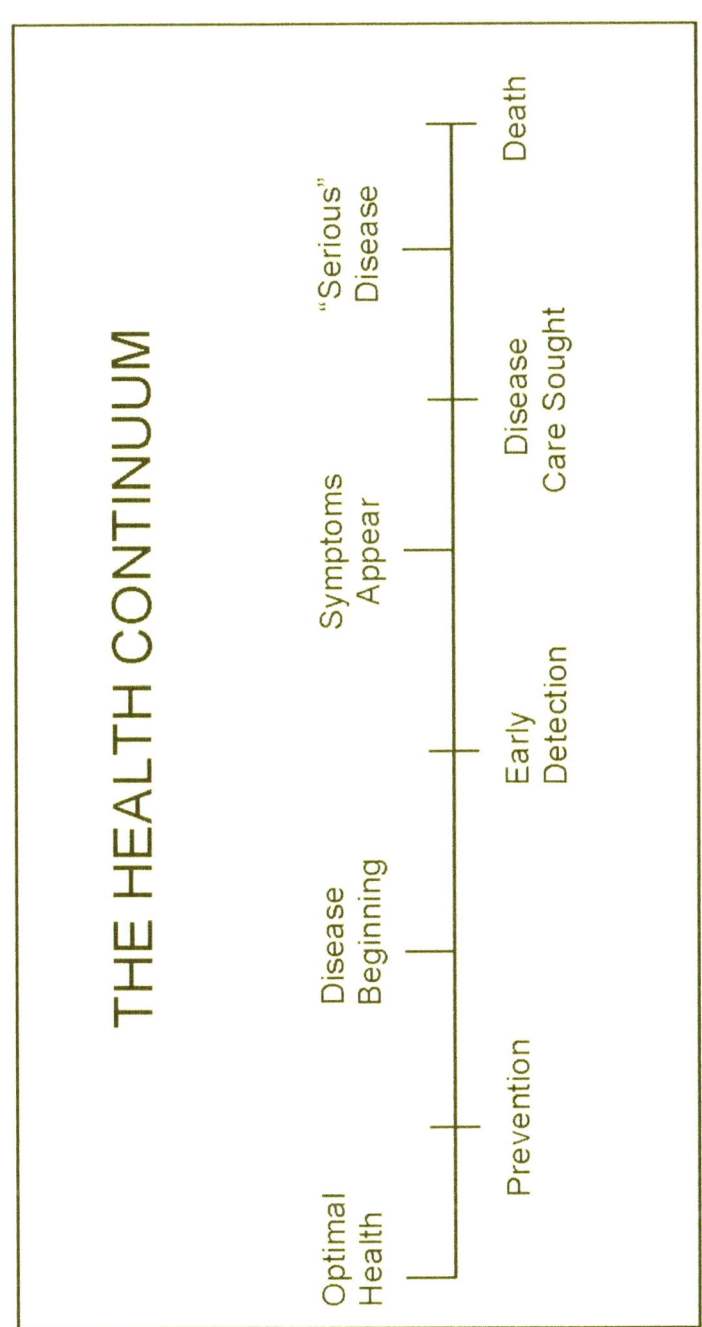

exercise, vitamins, chiropractic) actually prevents disease from beginning. **Early Detection** is any kind of test that simply discovers that disease has already begun. This would include things such as yearly medical exams, prostate exams and mammograms. While these serve their purpose, it is of key importance to understand the difference. Our current system sells early detection as prevention, which is absolutely wrong. Yes, it is nice to know that you have a disease sooner than later but this is not prevention (unless you have rationalized your belief such that you believe that you are preventing it from getting worse). Understand the difference because the time to practice a preventative lifestyle is before disease begins. Our system currently endorses a preventative lifestyle only after tests show that you didn't prevent disease in the first place.

Lastly, what most fail to understand is that there is a significant difference between **Optimal Health** and **Prevention**. Our current system believes that **Prevention** is the top level that we can achieve. We are told to practice a lifestyle such that we don't get heart disease or cancer or diabetes. While it is nice to prevent disease, this has absolutely nothing to do with the true definition of health. Recall that the actual definition of health goes out of its way to state that not having a disease does not mean that you're healthy. Health is about being the best that you can be to not only improve the quantity but also the quality of your life. It's not about not getting the bad stuff: it's about getting all the good stuff.

How does the Health Continuum apply to Alzheimer's?

You will discover in this book that almost all of the factors that contribute to Alzheimer's disease fit perfectly within the concept of the health continuum. The disease begins long before any symptoms appear and most wait until the disease has become serious before they do anything about it at which point it is usually far too late. There is a multitude of contributing factors and while many may think that singularly they're not important, together they slowly combine and progress over time.

More so, Alzheimer's is clinically broken up into 3 stages;

1. Pre-clinical
2. Mild Cognitive Impairment (MCI)
3. Dementia

On the Health Continuum these translate as:

Pre-clinical = Disease Beginning,

MCI = Symptoms Appears to Disease Care Sought

Dementia = Serious Disease

CHAPTER 6

SOCIETY'S PARADIGMS OF HEALTH

Do we know everything there is to know about health? Absolutely not. Do we know more than enough to be much healthier than we are? Absolutely yes! Then why are we not doing it?

How do we Choose our Health Decisions?

How do we choose our health decisions? The answer is twofold and both answers may surprise you. The first answer is that most people don't. They don't choose their health decisions because most people never decide. The word "decide" comes from the Latin decider, which literally means "to cut off all other possibilities". Hence, if we decide that we're going to eat healthy from now on, we actually do. If we decide that we're going to exercise regularly we actually do as we have cut off all other options. Unfortunately, most people decide to eat healthy, until they decide not to, in other words they go back to their old ways. If they had truly decided (cut off all other possibilities), there would be no going back.

The second way we choose is one of four options:

1. Knowledge
2. Fact
3. Truth
4. Belief

1. Knowledge

Very simply, some people know more than others and they will make their health choices based on what they know. If they don't know, they won't do. The problem when it comes to health, though, is that everyone thinks that they're an expert. Some are, in fact, resistant to learning anything new. (Do you know anyone like this?)

The demonstration I show in one of my workshops is where I take a glass and slowly start to fill it with water. The first few ounces represent what we learn in early childhood. The next few ounces are what we learn as a kid. The next few ounces are what we learn as a teenager. At this point the glass is almost full, which probably explains why teenagers think they already know it all. Now picture continuing to pour water in the glass as it begins to overflow and water starts to pour over the sides. Further move into adulthood and the water from the pitcher significantly overflows the glass and ends up in a puddle on the floor. (This could explain the phrase "you can't teach an old dog new tricks".) Then consider that some, if not a significant portion, of the water in the glass is simply wrong or certainly outdated information, especially when it comes to health. It is estimated that the field of knowledge in healthcare changes significantly every 3 to 4 years. You've also heard the saying "knowledge is power". The reality is that it's not knowledge that is power, rather it is *acting* on knowledge that is power.

2. Fact

Others will make their health decisions based on fact. "Just the facts, ma'am." They are the "scientific ones" who are looking for the **proven** health procedures and aren't interested in anything that hasn't been scientifically proven, feeling secure that science is on their side. (If you fall into this category, you will find my next chapter of interest.)

3. Truth

Still others make their health choices based on what they know to be the truth. It may not have been scientifically proven, it may not be common knowledge, but they know it to be true regardless of what others think. After all, it is said that new ideas go through 3 phases:

First – they are ridiculed

Second – they are violently opposed

Third – they are seen as self-evident

4. Belief

Or do we disregard knowledge, fact and truth and simply make our health choices on what we believe? "Not me", you say. Well again, after thousands of patients I have no doubt that we make our health choices based on what we believe.

Unfortunately, when it comes to Alzheimer's disease, most simply cross their fingers and hope. As you will discover, this needs to change.

> **Dr. Zielonka's Health Thought:**
> Do we know everything there is to know about health? Absolutely not.
> Do we know more than enough to be much healthier than we are? Absolutely yes!

Robert's Story

In hindsight, I really should have known something was wrong years earlier. I would forget the simplest of things on a more regular basis. I would forget birthdays and mix up my grandchildren's names. My wife would ask me to do things and they would completely slip my mind. At first, my family would make jokes about it but then the jokes came far too often for my liking.

As it happened more regularly, I finally gave in and went to see my doctor. Both she and I attributed it to stress and being overworked for which she prescribed an anti-depressant, told me to watch my stress and to reduce my work hours. That wasn't an option for me.

When it began to affect my work, I had to take it seriously. My job was very detail-oriented and I was responsible for the safety of others. At first, I would cope by writing everything down and delegating more of my duties. However, that became increasingly difficult and it certainly began to slow me down.

I was sure that others were beginning to notice and my constant reference to my notes for even the simplest of questions would be obvious to anyone. At this point I had to take a leave of absence (I never did return). I was fortunate enough that I had a decent pension and adequate savings as most people don't. To make matters worse, many insurance companies try to get out of paying disability benefits, especially if they believe you're just on "stress leave".

My new doctor arranged for a series of tests including a PET scan and spinal taps. Finally, a diagnosis of Alzheimer's disease.

I won't kid you – life has not been easy since then. I've tried 3 different drugs and my doctor says they're helping to slow the disease but how does one know? It's still progressing. I need help to do the simplest of tasks (including writing this) and I'm concerned not just for me but for the burden I've become on my family. I also fear that many of my friends will suffer the same fate if something isn't done.

I still remember the movie "The Notebook" as it is one of our favourites but it has a new meaning for us now. Is that my fate? Time will tell but I likely won't remember. Something must be done.

CHAPTER 7

WHY SCIENCE ISN'T SO SCIENTIFIC

Over the past twenty-seven years, I have provided care to thousands of patients, including a number of scientists and analysts. It has been my personal clinical experience - repeatedly I might add - that all of these scientists and analysts make a point of telling me that they make all of their health decisions "scientifically". Sounds reasonable, you say? I'd agree, except for the fact that it has also been my clinical experience that almost all of these same scientists and analysts end up making their health decisions anything but "scientifically". They use the same subjective opinions and sometimes false beliefs that are anything but "scientific". They may also utilize information that they believe is from scientific sources with no idea of just how biased that so-called scientific source may be. One example would be taking the FDA and Health Canada at face value without any understanding of just how many thousands have died from "safe and approved" drugs, only for those drugs to be recalled years later. Or just how frequently it is uncovered that these two government "authorities" are found to have what many actual experts describe as incestuous ties with various drug companies. If you believe that this is some type of conspiracy theory, then come up with reasonable answers to the following questions:

1. What scientific criteria were used that found a drug safe only to discover years later that the same drug was deadly?

2. How can one scientific study prove that a vitamin is beneficial while another scientific study proves that the exact same vitamin is not beneficial? More importantly, which do you choose to believe? Isn't the whole idea of "science" to remove the need for making decisions based on beliefs?

3. If the United States believes it has the best "science" in the world and if it believes that its healthcare system is solely based on the science, then why does the United States rank 37th in the world for healthcare? You must appreciate that double-blind studies have biases, and that assumes that they were conducted using sound protocols. One of the key questions that one must ask is, "Exactly what question was the study asking?" What do I mean? Try this. How many scientific studies have proven that cholesterol-lowering drugs save lives? The correct answer is zero. What cholesterol-lowering drug studies have shown is one thing and one thing only – that these drugs lower cholesterol. It is simply assumed that this saves lives. While this may be your belief, if

it were true why would a drug company not have a single scientific study to prove it?

How many scientific studies have proven that cholesterol-lowering drugs save lives? The correct answer is zero.

The best way to understand how unreasonable a double-blind randomized controlled scientific study could be based on the question being asked is best described in this analogy from well-known wellness expert Dr. James Chestnut:

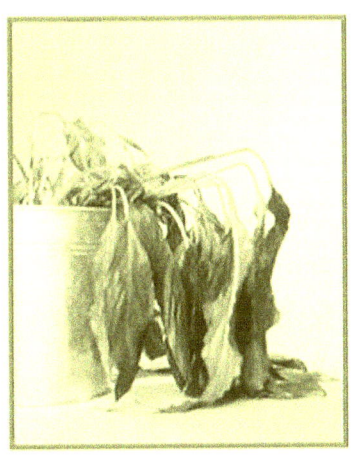

What would any reasonable person do for the above wilting plant? Water it, of course. But if I wanted to "prove" this "scientifically" in a double-blind randomized controlled study, I would need to take one hundred of these wilting plants and water them. I'd need to take another hundred wilting plants and give them a liquid that the plants thought was water but wasn't. Lastly, I would need to have another hundred wilting plants that I did nothing to.

And of course the person who then assessed how the plants reacted could not know what each plant received. So what's the problem, you ask? The problem is that you're assuming the obvious – that the wilting plants that actually received water all improved in their health. But what if in this example they didn't? What if after giving all these plants water they were still wilting? You would have a scientific double-blind randomized controlled study that could officially claim that water has no health benefit in making a wilting plant no longer wilt.

This could never happen, you say? Of course it could, because what if these same plants also all had soil that was completely devoid of any nutrients? Now the logical solution to help these plants would be to add nutrients to their soil. But to prove scientifically if this was beneficial for plants, again we would need to do our double-blind randomized controlled study. In this case, we would need our control group who received nothing, a group who got water and soil nutrients, a group who got water only, a group who got soil nutrients only, and groups who got a combination of placebo water and soil nutrients. But what if after doing all this, our water and soil nutrient plants were still wilting? Again, the drug company study would make headlines in the newspaper showing that vitamin X has been scientifically proven to have no benefit in helping disease Y. Oh, I'm sorry – we weren't talking about vitamins just yet? Alright – the newspaper headline would clearly - and accurately - I might add, state:

"New Scientific Study Shows That Water and Soil Nutrients Have No Health Benefits in Helping Wilting Plants Stop Wilting"

Couldn't happen, you say? Of course it could, because what if these same plants were all kept in a dark closet devoid of all sunlight? What many scientists and most of the general public fail to appreciate is that so-called scientific studies seek to answer a specific question and the question that is chosen can have a huge impact on just how useful the findings of that study actually are.

So what if we now do another double-blind randomized controlled study but this time with three variables, and all their placebo and control groups. Some plants received water, nutrients, and sunlight, some just water and sunlight but no nutrients, some with nutrients and sunlight but no water, etc. etc. And again, what if at the end our plants were still wilting? The newspaper headline would "accurately read" (according to the terms of the study):

"New Scientific Study Shows That Water, Nutrients, and Sunlight Have No Health Benefits in Helping Wilting Plants to Stop Wilting"

We of course know that such a finding is far from "accurate" as water, nutrients, and sunlight are essential for the health of any plant. (Try doing your own study where you stop giving these three things to your own plants and see what happens each and every time.) But according to the specific question being asked, our plants were still wilting. How is that possible, you say? Simple. All of the plants in question had gasoline poured into their soil. While you might think that this is an extreme example, appreciate that all living creatures, including both plants and humans, will always fail to function at optimal levels if they have deficiencies that are essential for life (water, nutrients, sunlight, vitamins) and/or if they are subjected to stressors or toxins (gasoline for the plants in our example, or a whole array of human stressors and toxins).

What's the logical bottom line? A study really can't disprove that a vitamin works, especially if numerous other studies have shown that it does work. And this doesn't even begin to touch on all the other factors missed (often purposely), such as using too small a quantity of vitamins, using the wrong form of vitamin, studying the subject for too short a period of time, or not using the required co-factors to ensure that the vitamin worked effectively - not to mention conflict of interest, faulty design and media bias. This is especially prevalent in many vitamin E and beta-carotene studies that have attempted to discredit their effectiveness. "Vitamin E Shown Not to Reduce Cardiovascular Disease" was the headline reported in the Journal of the American Medical Association (July 2005) in a study to test whether vitamin E supplementation decreased the risk of cardiovascular disease and cancer among healthy women. However, after reading the entire study it was found that for cardiovascular death there was a 24% reduction in risk! Why was the finding not heralded as a significant discovery? Because cardiovascular death was not one of the specific questions set up by the study.

In addition to asking the wrong question, there is another significant difference that is lost on most who live in the medical/drug world. There is a huge paradigm shift between those who live in the sick-care model of "health" and those who live in the health and wellness paradigm. The idea of using the methods in the sick-care model as an accurate way of measuring the health and wellness paradigm is completely invalid and defies common-sense. As scientist and world renowned supplementation expert Lyle MacWilliams states, "they're using the wrong yardstick". You cannot use a test that is designed to see if one drug has an effect on one reaction to then accurately gauge if a vitamin that works hand in hand with numerous other nutrients (not in isolation) can have the same effect on its own. As nutritional researcher Dr. Tim Wood states, "high doses of a single nutrient represent an incomplete and inappropriate approach to nutritional therapy…this would be analogous to testing the hypothesis that broccoli has cancer-preventative properties by putting people on a broccoli-only diet. It's not likely to work, and it carries the risk of creating severe nutrient imbalances, unwanted side effects, and misleading experimental artefacts."

Another way to put this into perspective would be to consider what would happen if we reversed the situation. What if we used the yardstick of the health and wellness paradigm to judge a drug from the sick-care paradigm? What would happen if we gave Lipitor or

Celebrex to a healthy child over the course of their lifetime? Would the results of such an experiment show that the child enjoyed a lifetime of health? Of course not – rather we would be jailed for child endangerment. Stop going to the sick-care experts and using their tools to judge your level of health. Your life depends on it. Stop believing that the sick care paradigm is superior as they believe they are. When it comes to health, nothing could be further from the truth.

What would happen if we gave Lipitor or Celebrex to a healthy child over the course of their lifetime?

People are entitled to have any belief that they choose. But as I explain to my patients, if I were to take you to the roof of my building and we both stepped off the ledge, it doesn't matter how many times you say "I don't believe in gravity" on the way down, we're still going to hit the ground.

Dr. Zielonka's Health Thought: "Believe in gravity."

Choose to believe in the numerous quality scientific studies listed in this book and the science of physiology and biochemistry that explains their rationale. Choose not to believe the few inaccurate "studies" that have ulterior motives or have chosen to ask the wrong question or come to the wrong conclusion. Follow this advice and you will experience a better quality and quantity of life.

CHAPTER 8

BRAIN HEALTH AND PRESCRIPTION DRUGS: WHY THIS APPROACH WON'T WORK

While there are certain prescription drugs that can save your life, the reality is that there is not a single drug on the market that doesn't have adverse side-effects, many of them serious and some of them deadly. More importantly, none of them understand the true definition of health. The hypocrisy of this approach when it comes to Alzheimer's disease is that there are drugs used to treat brain conditions and there are drugs that cause brain conditions.

Consider these facts:

- Every year 40,000 Canadians die from taking the "properly" prescribed drug in the "correct" dosage.
- 48% of Americans of all ages regularly take at least one prescription drug and 1 in 3 takes 2 or more prescription drugs.

- If you make it to 85 years of age, nearly 1 in 3 will be taking **10 or more** prescription drugs.
- 20% of children take at least one prescription drug.
- The US has 5% of the world's population yet takes 50% of the world's prescription drugs. It ranks 37th in the world for overall health. Can you name all of the other 36? By the way - Canada is 30th
- Did you know that drug companies spend more money on marketing than they do on research?
- Even with all these drugs, the average Canadian and American will spend the last 10 to 20 years of their lives in pain and suffering. Why would anyone want that?

So what does one do? As you would expect, my approach is both scientific and common sense. Many scientists hope that they will one day find a "cure" for many of these brain diseases. I would tell you that a "cure" and/or prevention already exists from a natural approach as you will discover. If an improved lifestyle and vitamin supplementation can optimize brain function and prevent disease without the need for drugs and their side-effects, then obviously that should be the approach. If drugs are necessary and the only alternative, lifestyle improvement and supplementation are still required.

Remember, there is currently no drug or vaccine that can cure, prevent or even slow Alzheimer's to any significant degree. Alzheimer's is always fatal.

Alzheimer's is always fatal

Let's be clear. I am talking about 2 things here: the drugs used by many for conditions other than brain health that are actually causative factors in the progression of Alzheimer's and those that are specifically designed for Alzheimer's yet ineffective.

How prescription drugs can actually cause Alzheimer's

Drugs can affect neurotransmitters and neuroplasticity in a number of ways:

- They can decrease the rate of synthesis of neurotransmitters by affecting the enzyme(s) required to make that neurotransmitter.
- They can either block or stimulate neurotransmitters.
- They can prevent neurotransmitter storage.
- They can prevent a neurotransmitter from binding to its receptor (known as receptor antagonists). These include drugs such as haloperidol, chlorpromazine, and clozapine to treat schizophrenia where they block dopamine.
- They can bind to a receptor and mimic the normal neurotransmitter. These are known as agonists such as Valium that mimics GABA to decrease anxiety.
- They can interfere with the deactivation of a neurotransmitter after it has been released prolonging its action.
- They can prevent an action potential from occurring.

Drugs that adversely affect brain health include:

- **Statins (cholesterol drugs)** – reduce cholesterol yet 25% of the dry weight of the brain is cholesterol. Cholesterol is also necessary to produce neurotransmitters as well as sex hormones, vitamin D and CoQ10. Even the FDA now requires statins to come with the warning of memory loss and confusion. Low cholesterol levels are also associated with an increased risk of dementia.

- **Tranquilizers** – such as Valium and Xanax prescribed for anxiety, insomnia and panic attacks actually cause mental confusion, depression, aggression and memory loss. Seniors who take these drugs increase their risk of dementia by 50%.

- **Antidepressants** – side-effects include anxiety attacks, hyperactivity, mood and behavioral changes, aggression, tremors, insomnia and even an increase in depression. Most importantly, they increase suicidal thoughts and do so most often in children, teenagers and young adults.

- **Sleeping Pills** – such as Ambien cause amnesia (Charlie Sheen called it the "Devil's Aspirin"). According to Dr. Kirk Parsley, former Navy Seal and sleep expert for the US Navy, EEGs show that people using drugs such as Ambien do not exhibit normal sleep patterns; rather their patterns resemble those in a coma. According to Dr. Parsley, "taking a sleeping pill does not put you to sleep; it renders you unconscious, thus bypassing the restorative value of sleep. This is disastrous for your brain since it's during sleep that your brain consolidates the day's memories, clears itself of metabolic debris, maintains and repairs itself, and grows new cells."

- **Anticholinergic drugs** – Given that acetylcholine is a neurotransmitter involved in learning and memory, any drug that reduces acetylcholine would obviously negatively affect these abilities. These drugs cause mental confusion, incoherent speech, memory loss, hallucinations and other symptoms that resemble dementia. Given that dementia and Alzheimer's are associated with low acetylcholine levels, this should come as no surprise.
- **Over The Counter drugs (OTCs)** - used for cold remedies, allergies, headache, cough, sinus, motion sickness, insomnia and acid-reflux problems are also anticholinergic.

The above list is by no means exhaustive. Your goal should be to minimize prescription drugs wherever possible, seek natural and effective alternatives and certainly be aware of all the side-effects of any prescription drug you may be taking. Better yet, by living a lifetime of health, one can often avoid any need for drugs in the first place.

Drugs for Alzheimer's Disease:

These are primarily acetylcholinesterase inhibitors, which reduce the rate of acetylcholine breakdown. It is important to note here that these drugs slow down the breakdown of the neurotransmitter acetylcholine – they do not increase the production of it.

1. Donepezil (*Aricept*)
2. Galantamine (*Razadyne*)
3. Rivastigmine (*Exelon* and *Exelon Patch*)

Aricept works as a cholinesterase inhibitor preventing the enzyme cholinesterase from breaking down acetylcholine but doesn't stop the disease from advancing and actually triggers the production of more cholinesterase (this can be dangerous if the drug is stopped suddenly). Side-effects include headache, nausea, vomiting, loss of appetite, diarrhea, joint pain, drowsiness and slowed heart rate.

Memantine belongs to the group of drugs known as *NMDA* (N-methyl-D-aspartate) *receptor antagonists*. It does not cure Alzheimer's disease but it is used to decrease symptoms. It works in the brain by blocking the effect of chemicals that cause symptoms of Alzheimer's disease such as decreased memory and other mental functions. It also prevents the transmission necessary to create memories.

Neither deal with the root cause nor can they stop progression of the disease.

Common Side-Effects:

- Nausea and vomiting (10-20% of users) – this is linked to cholinergic excess (cholinergic syndrome) with increased acetylcholine throughout the body and parasympathetic discharge.

Less Common Side-Effects:

- Muscle cramps
- Bradycardia
- Decreased appetite and weight
- Increased gastric acid production
- Tearing
- Increased salivation

CHAPTER 9

THE 3 BIGGEST REASONS SOCIETY HAS IT WRONG THE 17-YEAR PROBLEM

Let's get right to the point and the $64,000 question. How is it that Alzheimer's and other forms of dementia cost the United States $277 billion last year yet I have the answer? Here are the 3 biggest reasons where society has been misled and why we have it so wrong.

1. **The Wrong Cause** – It was way back in 1906 that Dr. Alois Alzheimer examined the brain post mortem of a German woman named Auguste Deter who died from dementia in her fifties after being under the care of Dr. Alzheimer for 5 years. Dissection of her brain revealed protein plaques and neural tangles that had not been seen before as well as cortex atrophy. It was not until 1984 that the plaques were identified as beta amyloid and 1986 that the tangles were identified as tau proteins. The conclusion? It must be the amyloid plaques that were responsible for the dementia and as such, for over the

past century, there has not been a single drug that has been successful at curing Alzheimer's by removing this plaque.

2. **The Wrong Approach** – Obviously if we have the wrong cause we must be taking the wrong approach. Furthermore, society has been led to believe that there is one drug for every disease and sure, if you want to try anything else it might be a little helpful. This couldn't be further from the truth. Both health and disease involve a multitude of factors that are also interdependent on one another. We must also take into account that these factors will affect different people differently under certain circumstances and as such each person may require a different approach.

Remember that glass of water I talked about in chapter 1? Let's make it a bucket and let's think of the water as being your reservoir of health. If every health problem only ever involved one hole in your bucket, then all you'd have to do is plug that one hole. Health doesn't work that way. Most health problems involve numerous different contributing factors. Picture that same bucket with 8 holes in it and how you'd be losing your water and reservoir of health. You need to plug all the holes to be successful – in other words – one drug for one hole will never solve the problem. By the way, in the case of Alzheimer's, at least 36 different factors have now been identified as contributing to its development and progression with varying degrees of importance specific to each individual. You might have factors 1, 2, 6, 9, 12, 24 and 32 whereas your spouse may have 7, 8, 3, 22, 19, 12, 20, 5 and 10 in that order of priority. One drug will never fix that.

3. **Way Too Slow** – So if the solution is science-based, why isn't every doctor aware of it? Good question. I can't tell you the number of times I've read a front page newspaper story or lead television news segment on a "breaking" health topic that was something I spoke about in a health lecture 15-20 years ago. How is that possible?

Here's how. In 2001, the National Academy of Medicine, then known as the Institute of Medicine, published a landmark study that found there was a lag of **17 years** between when health scientists learn something significant from rigorous scientific research and when health practitioners change their patient care to reflect that new research. That's right – our "health-care" system is 17 years behind the times and not surprisingly, this study was published 17 years ago. To prevent Alzheimer's, you don't have 17 years to wait. By following the simple 7-step program in this book you won't have to.

There is a lag of 17 years between when health scientists learn something significant from rigorous scientific research and when health practitioners change their patient care to reflect that new research

CHAPTER 10

DR. Z'S 12 BIG IDEAS YOU NEED TO UNDERSTAND AND ACCEPT ABOUT HEALTH

1. **"Health"** - As discussed in Chapter 4, health is the optimal state. The primary reason this is so difficult for many to understand and achieve is because society has been sadly misled to believe otherwise and has built a system that focuses on pain, symptoms and "managing" disease, usually through artificial means. The second reason that it is difficult for many to appreciate is that, while people say they accept this definition, few are willing to take the daily actions to achieve it.

2. **"Health Continuum"** – Please review Chapter 4 in depth. Again, many people say they understand this concept but then equate prevention and early detection as one and the same or health and prevention as one and the same. They are not. This concept easily explains people's different attitudes towards

health. Will one french fry kill you? No. Will a lifetime of nothing but french fries lead you to an early grave? Of course. Will missing one workout hurt you? Probably not. Will never exercising throughout your entire life have a negative impact? Of course. Will a brief exposure to one toxin hurt you? You'll survive. Will exposure to a lifetime of carcinogens and pesticides have serious consequences whether or not you know this is happening? Highly likely, and of course this will vary depending on your particular biological make-up.

This is why some will take measures over the course of their lifetime to minimize these while others will laugh it off saying we all have to die sometime. You get to choose: are you someone who takes action when the arteries to your heart are clogged 10% or do you wait until they're clogged 90%? The reverse is also true. Don't expect a vitamin to rebuild tissue overnight. Are you going to let your brain slowly and prematurely degenerate over the course of your lifetime with less than optimal function or are you going to take the action steps to keep your dimmer switch at 100%?

3. **Power** - as in you have the power to control your health and destiny more than you have been led to believe. It does require knowledge and effort on your part. You must take the appropriate action over the course of your lifetime.

4. **The Brain is...** - For some bizarre reason we appreciate that we can do things to keep our body healthy or our heart healthy

but fail to realize that the same is true for our brain. Your brain is like any other organ: by taking the right steps over the course of your lifetime you can maximize your brain function, prevent most degenerative diseases and maximize both performance and function.

5. **Your Thoughts** – are under your control and have far more of an impact than you were ever led to believe. You're entitled to any belief you choose; just appreciate that those beliefs have consequences whether you believe them or not.

6. **Chemical Pathways** – Physiological processes in your body work along very specific chemical pathways. Many vitamins used for the management or prevention of disease work along the exact same chemical pathway as does the prescription drug designed for the same disease. Often, the only difference is far fewer side-effects and just as good efficiency - if not better. Furthermore, vitamins work along chemical pathways that drugs cannot achieve: – they work along chemical pathways that achieve and maintain optimum health and optimum function.

7. **Hope is nice…** - In my health centre one of the many sayings I have coined over the years is "Hope is nice but action is better". A lifetime of health requires a lifetime of healthy actions.

8. **There will always be deniers** – For many reasons there will always be those who will spend more time arguing about the

value of health and try to disprove healthy steps than actually taking action on their health and will try to convince you likewise. Whether it's confirmation bias (selectively choosing the research that supports your beliefs while dismissing any that contradicts your position), arrogance, ignorance, ulterior motives, dogma, emotions, monetary gain, laziness or simply being closed-minded and stuck in old paradigms, their rationale and excuses will continue. Be aware that this may include skewed science, significant dogma and serious financial motives that attempt to brainwash society as a whole. Never let these people deter you from taking the common sense and logical approach to health where you will reap the rewards over a lifetime.

9. **The Five Keys** – Your body and mind work as a whole. Unlike our sick-care system that focuses on one drug for one specific symptom, your body and brain require an overall comprehensive approach to target all the factors involved and all the factors required for optimal health. Follow all five of The 5 Keys to Health over the course of your lifetime.

10. **The Big Picture Approach** - This concept was first described in my book *Health Beliefs – Deadly Choices*. Similar to the Five Keys to Health, you must appreciate that most "health conditions" require a multifactorial approach whereas the drug approach is more geared towards one drug for one

symptom. Even beyond drugs, many still fail at recovery by only trying one thing at a time. If you have seven different factors contributing to your illness, then you must address all seven at the same time.

11. **"Vitamins work** – the only requirement is that you actually take them".

12. **Your body has an innate wisdom** – As a functional health doctor and award winning neuro-functional chiropractor, I am a bigger "believer" than most that your body has an incredible ability to not only heal itself but to adapt to a changing environment. I would further state that it goes beyond being a "believer"; rather I know it to be fact. Some would then ask if the body is so wise, why does disease progress? It does so because most go out of their way with a lifetime of poor health habits in a nasty environment under chronic stress to destroy it. When the body adapts, it is doing so in response to these conditions. As you will discover shortly in this book, this becomes extremely important with respect to the cause of and the cure for Alzheimer's disease.

PART THREE

YOUR BRAIN AND ALZHEIMER'S

CHAPTER 11

HOW THE BRAIN WORKS: NEURONS, NEUROPLASTICITY AND NEUROTRANSMITTERS

Growing up you may have been led to believe that the heart was the most important organ in your body and I'm sure most cardiovascular surgeons would agree. But without a doubt, the master system in the body is your brain and the accompanying nervous system by which it transmits its messages to the rest of the body. Your brain controls everything. It is responsible for not only conscious thought, mood and emotion but also the control of every cell, tissue and organ in the body. Let's not forget healing, repair, self-regulation and so much more. Why on earth then, would we not want to provide it with the nutrients it needs and maintain it at an optimal level of function?

Here are some terms that are important to understand:

Neurons: These are your brain cells. Surprisingly, however, unknown to most you will discover that you also have neurons in your gut.

Neuroplasticity: This is the brain's ability to form new neural connections to reorganize itself after injury or disease. Thus, neurons can adjust their activities in response to new situations and changes in their environment. There was a time when we thought the brain was not capable of doing this. We now know that the brain is indeed capable of significant change and adaptability. Alzheimer's is essentially a dysfunction in neuroplasticity caused by a multitude of factors.

Neurotransmitters: These are substances that transmit messages from one brain cell to another. I have also included the chemical structure of each to convey the idea that as chemical compounds they can be altered or affected by, or react with, other substances. The following are the main neurotransmitters in the brain:

1. **Dopamine** – Best known for feelings of pleasure (known as the pleasure neurotransmitter), dopamine is also involved in motivation, addiction, and movement. Given its involvement in movement, a lack of dopamine can actually lead to Parkinson's disease causing involuntary shaking of the hands and difficulty walking.

2. **Serotonin** – This neurotransmitter contributes to happiness and well-being (hence known as the happiness or mood neurotransmitter). This is also the neurotransmitter most often associated with depression when levels are not adequate. Antidepressant drugs (SSRIs) are designed to target serotonin and make it more available in the brain. While it is manufactured in the brain, 90% of the serotonin supply is found in the digestive tract. It also aids in both your sleep cycle and digestive system function. It can be affected by both light exposure and exercise.

3. **Endorphins** – Known as the euphoria neurotransmitter, it is released during exercise, excitement and sex. It produces a sense of euphoria, well-being and pain reduction similar to the effect of drugs like morphine and codeine without the addiction or dependence.

4. **Adrenaline** – This neurotransmitter (known as the 'fight or flight' or stress neurotransmitter) is produced during times of stress and excitement. As such, it increases heart rate and awareness. **Epinephrine** is the more scientifically accepted name for **adrenaline**.

5. **Noradrenaline** - This neurotransmitter is also involved in the 'fight or flight' syndrome and in improving your concentration (hence known as the concentration neurotransmitter). One of its main effects is on attention where low levels are linked to ADHD. When a stress response has been activated, it can affect

your heart rate, blood sugar, and blood flow to muscles. It is also known as **Norepinephrine**.

6. **Acetylcholine** - This neurotransmitter is involved in learning, thought and memory (hence known as the learning neurotransmitter). It is associated with attention, awakening and the activation of muscle.

7. **Glutamate** - This is the most common brain neurotransmitter and is also involved in learning and memory (known as the memory neurotransmitter). It is also involved in the creation of nerve contacts. Approximately half of brain synapses involve glutamate.

[Chemical structure of glutamate]

8. **GABA** – It calms the nerves in the central nervous system (hence known as the calming neurotransmitter) and helps with motor control and vision. High levels lead to increased focus while low levels lead to increased anxiety.

[Chemical structure of GABA]

Glutamate and GABA work hand in hand to balance excitement levels in the brain. GABA is "inhibitory" and glutamate is "excitatory". Substance abuse can change the balance of these neurotransmitters, for example, alcohol decreases glutamate and increases GABA while tranquilizers increase GABA activity.

As you will discover in the following chapters, by knowing which neurotransmitters are involved in which functions, we can alter the function and reactions that occur in the brain and the body with specific vitamin supplementation.

Health Fact #3:

More people die from Alzheimer's than from breast cancer and prostate cancer combined.

CHAPTER 12

IS THE NIGHTMARE INEVITABLE? THE ADVANCED VERSION

By this point in the book you've done two things: 1) you've flipped your coin and decided you're going to take action to prevent heart disease or cancer from ever happening, and 2) you've accepted that your brain is no different and that Alzheimer's and dementia can also be prevented in most cases.

Alzheimer's disease is currently the 6th leading cause of death in the United States affecting over 5 million Americans. What's worse is that if you plan on living to 85, you're back to flipping that coin as nearly half of the population (47%) will be affected by Alzheimer's. What that means is that if you have a spouse, either you or they will suffer from Alzheimer's. Even worse, it is really the only cause of death among the top 10 in the United States where medical treatments are unable to prevent or slow the progression of the disease to any appreciable degree. Alzheimer's is always fatal.

If you plan to live past 85, either you or your spouse will suffer from Alzheimer's. The other one will be the caretaker.

Why Do People Die from Alzheimer's?

Although Alzheimer's disease shortens people's life spans, it is usually not the **direct** cause of a person's death. Rather, people die from complications from the illness. The actual death of a person with Alzheimer's may be caused by another condition due to their frailness as the disease progresses. Their ability to cope with infection and other physical problems will be impaired due to the progression of the dementia.

Further, one forgets the most basic of activities, including self-care, and the body eventually shuts down as the condition progresses.

What Exactly is Alzheimer's?

Alzheimer's is a progressive neurological disease affecting memory and thought with the following hallmark features:

1. Decreased production of the neurotransmitter acetylcholine
2. Free radical damage to brain cells
3. Beta-amyloid protein plaque build-up
4. Neurofibrillary tangles

5. Loss of insulin (and IGF-1) receptor and signaling on neuron membranes
6. Shrinkage of the prefrontal cortex and hippocampus as well as enlarged ventricles

The two Classifications

There are two main classifications of Alzheimer's: **Early Onset** and **Late Onset**.

Early Onset can occur as early as your 30s and can have a genetic component of gene mutation as we will discuss shortly. It is important to understand two key factors with respect to Early Onset Alzheimer's:

1) Early Onset only accounts for 10% of Alzheimer's cases

2) even if you have this gene mutation it is not inevitable that this gene will be expressed provided you take the necessary lifestyle steps that control whether this gene will be expressed or not.

This is the field of epigenetics where science now understands that simply having a genetic predisposition does not mean it has to happen. The bigger determining factor is whether or not that gene is turned on or off, which can be greatly influenced by living a healthy lifestyle and taking all of the necessary steps as outlined in this book.

Late Onset Alzheimer's accounts for 90% of Alzheimer's cases and is greatly linked to dietary and lifestyle factors. While there is no specific gene that causes Late Onset Alzheimer's, there is a genetic risk factor known as the apolipoprotein E-4 (APOE ε4 gene). However, again it is important to note that there are many with this genetic risk factor that never develop Alzheimer's and others that do who don't have this genetic risk factor.

The Seven Stages of Alzheimer's

The most common classification from a timeline perspective is to place the progression of Alzheimer's into seven stages as follows;

Stage 1: No Impairment
There are absolutely no symptoms of Alzheimer's even though the disease process has started.

Stage 2: Very Mild Decline
Minor memory problems are noted which are almost always attributed to age or stress, often even joked about. The person will still do well on standard memory tests and neither family nor doctor is likely to suspect that anything is wrong.

Stage 3: Mild Decline
Family members may begin to notice cognitive problems. This may include finding the right word during conversations, remembering names of new acquaintances and losing personal possessions.

Stage 4: Moderate Decline
Symptoms of Alzheimer's are now apparent, including having difficulty with simple arithmetic, poor short-term memory, an inability to manage finances and forgetting details about their life. Sadly, this is usually the stage when Alzheimer's is first diagnosed.

Stage 5: Moderately Severe Decline

At this stage people will begin to need help with many day-to-day activities including getting dressed. The inability to recall simple details about themselves and significant confusion are prevalent. They can still maintain functionality such as bathing and using the toilet. They usually know their family members.

Stage 6: Severe Decline

Constant supervision is necessary, usually of a professional nature. Symptoms include confusion, unawareness of their surroundings, an inability to recognize faces except for their closest friends and family, loss of bladder and bowel control, major personality changes and behavioral problems, wandering and the need for assistance with toileting and bathing.

Stages 7: Very Severe Decline

This is the final stage of Alzheimer's and they are near death. People lose the ability to communicate and may eventually lose their ability to swallow.

Although the process of Alzheimer's began at least 20 years prior, on average most people live between four and eight years following diagnosis.

CHAPTER 13

THE THREE THEORIES OF ALZHEIMER'S... AND WHY THEY'RE WRONG

There are three main theories accepted by the vast majority of the medical community as to the mechanism of Alzheimer's, dementia and age-related memory loss.

1. **The Cholinergic Hypothesis** – Alzheimer's is caused by the reduced synthesis of the neurotransmitter acetylcholine. Since most people experience a decrease in acetylcholine after age 55 (due to decreased brain accessibility to choline, which is necessary to make acetylcholine), the likelihood of Alzheimer's increases. The most commonly used Alzheimer's drugs attempt to address this issue, however; they are not very effective in the long run as their mechanism of action doesn't boost acetylcholine production, rather; it only attempts to prevent its breakdown.

2. **Beta-amyloid protein plaque build-up -** A substance known as Amyloid precursor protein (APP) is critical to neuron growth, neuron survival and post-injury repair. However, in Alzheimer's, APP gets divided into smaller fragments by enzymes that produce beta-amyloid fibrils and form clumps. This amyloid plaque causes free radical damage and inflammation to nerve cells, which damages brain cells and accelerates Alzheimer's progression.

3. **Tau Hypothesis** – To simplify, a protein known as Tau protein experiences abnormal pairing with other threads of tau proteins and forms neurofibrillary tangles inside the nerve cell bodies. This causes the microtubules to disintegrate and collapses the neuron's transport system. This results in disrupted communication between nerve cells and eventually in cell death.

So Why is this Wrong?

It's not necessarily that these three theories are wrong, in fact they do happen, but rather they're not **the cause** of Alzheimer's. This explains why all the drugs that have been developed over the years have failed miserably. It has been over 100 years since Alzheimer's was discovered and there is still no cure.

The good news is that there are some scientists who have begun to question these theories and whether they're correct. The bad news is that there are other doctors who believe that it's not that the current drugs don't work but rather that they're given too late after the disease has progressed too far. They would like to see the same drugs given much earlier to all. Needless to say I don't subscribe to that approach.

Remember, as discussed in chapter 10, your body has an innate wisdom with the incredible ability to not only heal itself but to adapt to a changing environment. Given that, doesn't it make sense that the plaque build-up is not the cause of the disease but rather the body's response to protect brain cells from infection, toxins and inflammation? This would also explain why drugs that target removal of the beta-amyloid plaque have been so unsuccessful. In fact, a study published just this year from Harvard Medical School showed that beta-amyloid protein actually protects the brain from the effects of the herpes virus.

Plaque build-up is not the cause of the disease but rather the body's response to protect brain cells from infection, toxins and inflammation

Therefore, beta-amyloid build-up is the body's natural defense to a brain under assault from inflammation, sub-optimal nutrients and toxic exposures. Further proving this point is the fact that there are documented cases of cognitive decline in people who have no beta-amyloid plaque build-up and people with beta-amyloid plaque build-up who have no cognitive decline.

Progressive scientists now look to the fragmentation of the APP that is critical to neuron growth, neuron survival and post-injury repair as the mechanism of Alzheimer's. When APP gets divided into smaller fragments Alzheimer's is likely to progress. When APP is only divided into 2 fragments, optimal function is maintained.

As such, Alzheimer's is not about beta-amyloid plaques and Tau proteins but rather this fragmentation of the APP and at last count at least 36 different factors that influence that fragmentation, including inflammation, toxins, blood sugar, vitamin deficiency, hormone imbalances, stress, vascular issues and trauma.

Health Fact #4:

Twice as many women die from Alzheimer's as do men.

CHAPTER 14

WHICH MEANS THE TESTING IS WRONG AS WELL

"My husband is seeing the specialist at the hospital next week about his memory loss. Last week he forgot where he lived and got lost on the way home. The doctor is one of the top specialists and deals with lots of Alzheimer's cases so we're hopeful".

Well that's unfortunate… and that's unfortunate, for many reasons;

1. It's unfortunate that your husband forgot how to get home. That's a serious sign – not just a lapse in memory or that he was under stress.

2. It's nice that you're hopeful but to be blunt hope counts for nothing. And unfortunately, you're entering a system that really understands little about Alzheimer's. You now know that they're 17 years behind and that they're taking the wrong approach because they have the wrong theory on what causes Alzheimer's in the first place. Add to this that this process

started 20 years before getting to this point. All of these facts add up to why this "specialist" sees so many Alzheimer's patients.

3. Worse yet, chances are the tests that they'll perform, as well-meaning as these doctors may be, will pretty much be useless. They are likely to be the most well-known cognitive tests including the MOCA (Montreal Cognitive Assessment) and MMSE (Mini Mental State Examination) as well as "advanced" testing including MRIs and PET scans. So why are they useless? Here's why.

The MOCA is comprised of questions such as recognizing the drawing of a lion, camel and rhinoceros and drawing the hands on a clock representing 11:10. The MMSE includes questions such as reading the phrase "close your eyes" on a page and then following that instruction. Both tests include recalling items, counting backwards from 100 by 7, and knowing the day, month and year as well as the city that you're in. By the time you're diagnosed with failing these questions your disease has progressed way too far.

As for the MRIs and PET scans, they're still looking for beta-amyloid plaque, which a) isn't the cause of the problem and b) has progressed way too far.

If they have the wrong theory and hence are doing the wrong testing way too late, how on earth can they ever solve the problem? In most cases this process began 20 years ago and will progress through 7 different stages. Sadly, most Alzheimer's patients are not diagnosed until stage 4.

One needs to think of Alzheimer's not so much as a disease but rather a neuro-protective reaction to a brain under assault through decades of less than optimal brain health. One also needs to appreciate that becoming forgetful with age is **not** a normal process of aging, contrary to popular belief and that of our sick-care system.

As we will discuss, specialized functional health doctors utilize entirely different testing and a completely different approach.

CHAPTER 15

THE SIX TYPES OF ALZHEIMER'S

These factors categorize into six main categories. It is important to note that your particular cause of Alzheimer's is likely to be a combination of the following six types:

1. **Inflammatory** – This is characterized by increased inflammatory markers and shrinkage of the hippocampus. To correct this, one must seek the cause of the inflammation (poor diet, leaky gut, infection, oral hygiene, etc. or a combination thereof) rather than just take drugs to reduce the inflammation.

2. **Atrophic amnestic** – A deficiency of adequate trophic support (vitamins, minerals, hormones, BDNF – Brain-Derived Neurotrophic Factor), whether rapid or prolonged, will adversely affect normal brain function. This deficiency is increased in the elderly due to poor absorption of the necessary vitamins as a result of decreased stomach acid.

3. **Toxic** – whether through mercury and aluminum from exposure to dental fillings, vaccines and even the consumption of fish, pollution in the atmosphere and water or bio-toxins from mold and Lyme disease, our brains have accumulated a lifetime of toxins. Add exposure from cleaning products, pesticides, cosmetics and more which progresses over a lifetime as per the theory of the health continuum affects individuals differently depending on their susceptibility.

4. **Glycotoxic** – Poorly regulated blood sugar doesn't just disrupt normal insulin function and lead to type 2 and type 3 diabetes, it also results in advanced glycation end products (AGE – think of your cells as being sugar coated), and shrinkage of the brain.

5. **Trauma** – to be discussed in chapter 20.

6. **Vascular** – Think of vascular insufficiency to the brain as similar to what happens during stroke – a resultant lack of oxygen and required nutrients. This is also seen in those suffering from sleep apnea as one literally stops breathing during their sleep.

Brain Shrinkage

Since Alzheimer's results in cell death, your brain will actually shrink in size. Shrinkage occurs to both the prefrontal cortex and the hippocampus. The prefrontal cortex is responsible for personality expression, decision-making, social behavior and planning complex cognitive behavior. The hippocampus is the area of the brain that is mainly responsible for memory as well as emotions and motivation.

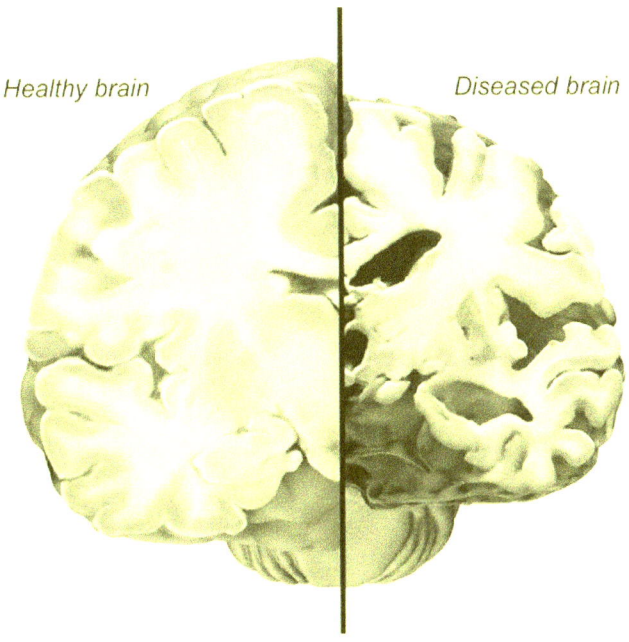

CHAPTER 16

THE ROLE OF GENETICS

Does genetics play a big role in Alzheimer's? The correct answer is a big yes AND a big no. Please let me explain in detail because this is extremely important to understand.

If you've been a regular attendee of my Human Performance Health Series over the years or a subscriber to my new podcast *The Science of Brain Health*, you may know that I have some of the worst genes in the world. You could literally go from head to toe on my late father with serious health issues, including heart disease, diabetes, osteoporosis, osteoarthritis, diverticulitis, skin cancer, colon cancer, lung cancer and more. As for my mom, it's diabetes, cancer, osteoarthritis, osteoporosis and more. If genetics was the sole factor, I might just as well give up now. The good news is that I, and so should you, realize that epigenetics plays a far larger role in your health.

> **Do genetics play a big role in Alzheimer's?**
> **The correct answer is a big yes AND a big no.**

What is epigenetics? It's the field of science that deals with the factors that influence whether the particular genes you have are actually expressed or not. You should understand that just because you have genes that may not be great, that doesn't mean that it has to be a self-fulfilling prophecy. And what determines if a particular gene is expressed? It's your lifestyle. That's right; all the factors we discuss in this book can help you prevent Alzheimer's, not to mention keep you healthier overall, regardless of your genetics.

Contrary to medical dogma, epigenetics is always more important than genetics

It's important to understand the above, because now that you appreciate the importance of epigenetics, the one place genetics makes a big difference is in the *possible* development of Alzheimer's. Let me explain.

Of your 23 pairs of chromosomes, there is a percentage of the population that have a gene variant on chromosome 19 known as ApoE4. Apo is an abbreviation for Apolipoprotein, which is a protein that carries fat.

If you have zero copies of this variant passed down from your parents, then you have a 9% chance of ending up with Alzheimer's. However, if you have one copy of this variant passed on from either parent (known as heterozygous), your odds now jump to 30%. It is estimated that 25% of white Americans and 33% of African Americans carry one copy. If you have two copies (one from each parent known as homozygous) your lifetime odds jump to 50 to 90%.

What does this all mean and what should you do? Some are so scared that they simply don't want to know and actually refuse to be tested. I would advise two things:

1. you should always know and then take the appropriate steps – get tested.

2. even if you have 2 copies of this variant, it does **not** make it inevitable that you will contract Alzheimer's, rather it's all the more reason you should follow my Simple 7-step Solution to Prevent the Nightmare of Alzheimer's in this book beginning today.

CHAPTER 17
TYPE 3 DIABETES

You are likely well aware that diabetes influences many other health issues. You can add Alzheimer's to that list. The groundbreaking Rotterdam study looked at 6,370 subjects over more than 2 years and found that Type 2 diabetes doubled the risk of a patient having dementia while patients on insulin had four times the risk.

The term type 3 diabetes was coined in 2005 when a team of researchers examining post-mortem brain tissue found that Alzheimer's may be a neuroendocrine disease associated with insulin signaling. The team coined the term type 3 diabetes because it has elements of both type 1 and type 2 diabetes: there is a decrease in the production of insulin and there is a resistance to insulin receptors.

Alzheimer's is characterized by both low insulin levels and insulin resistance within the central nervous system as opposed to type 2 diabetes, which is characterized by high insulin levels and insulin resistance outside the central nervous system. Both insulin resistance and hyperinsulinemia cause a reduction in brain insulin.

Insulin receptors are found in areas of the brain that are responsible for cognition. Insulin activates pathways associated with learning and long-term memory. Insulin also helps to regulate processes such as neuron survival, energy metabolism, and brain plasticity, which are required for learning and memory. If there is peripheral insulin resistance then cognition will be negatively affected.

In addition to regulating blood sugar levels, insulin also functions as a growth factor for all cells, including neurons in the brain. Insulin is required to support Tau protein and microtubule integrity. Thus, a lack of brain insulin contributes to beta-amyloid plaque and neurofibrillary tangle synthesis in Alzheimer's.

When insulin levels reach an exceedingly high level in the blood, the beta-amyloid peptide is modulated. Exaggerated elevation of plasma insulin levels causes amyloid peptide levels in the cerebrospinal fluid to increase, which adversely affects memory.

Advanced glycation end products are found in higher concentrations in both hyperglycemia and Alzheimer's contributing to both oxidative stress and nerve cell damage.

As such, it is important to keep your fasting blood sugar (glucose) level below 5.0 mmol/L (90 mg/dL). One reason for this is the fact that there is an enzyme in the brain that breaks down both insulin and amyloid plaque. In cases where insulin levels are high, the brain enzyme is so busy breaking down insulin that it allows amyloid plaque to build up. High levels of amyloid plaque (also known as beta-amyloid protein) essentially strangle brain cells from the outside and generate significant amounts of free radicals that further damage brain cell structure and function. High blood sugar also increases brain inflammation, which contributes to Alzheimer's disease development.

Health Fact #5:

Having Type 2 Diabetes doubles your risk of Alzheimer's and other forms of dementia. Being on insulin quadruples it.

CHAPTER 18

CHRONIC BRAIN INFLAMMATION

Science now knows that chronic inflammation plays a major role in most disease and certainly does so in Alzheimer's disease. As such, reducing inflammation is of key importance in both preventing Alzheimer's and achieving optimal health. This can be achieved through proper diet, proper supplementation, regular exercise and avoiding injury. Seven ways to achieve this are as follows:

1. **Eat fat** – Contrary to what many were led to believe with respect to nutrition, good fat is not the culprit. Monounsaturated fats such as extra virgin olive oil, saturated fats such as coconut oil, medium chain triglycerides (MCTs) and short chain triglycerides (SCTs), and especially essential fatty acids (EFAs) are all necessary for proper brain function and health.

2. **Minimize excessive carbohydrates** – The SAD diet (the standard American diet) is terrible for health and a significant factor in causing inflammation. It literally sugar-coats cells

and feeds yeast, and of course disrupts insulin balance leading to diabetes.

3. **Maintain healthy blood sugar levels** – Similar to #2, this is why some refer to Alzheimer's as Type 3 diabetes.

4. **Exercise** – Regular exercise is key for many reasons, including maintaining muscle mass, optimal blood flow and optimal lymphatic drainage, all factors in reducing inflammation.

5. **Avoid drugs that destroy health** – As you have already read about in this book and what I wrote about at length in my book *The Science of Vitamins Meets Optimum Health and Common Sense*, there are many prescription and over-the-counter drugs that have significant adverse effects on your health and are causative factors in both inflammation and Alzheimer's. These include statins, metformin, antacids, antidepressants and more.

6. **Stop grain** – No, this is not just a preference to annoy servers in restaurants. Grain leads to leaky gut, may contain mold and myotoxins, adversely affects your microbiome and is typically high in omega 6 fatty acids, all of which have adverse health effects, cause inflammation, and are significant factors in the development and progression of Alzheimer's.

7. **Practice safe participation** in sports to lessen the risk of trauma and brain injury.

Health Fact #6:

From the year 2000 to 2015, deaths from Alzheimer's climbed 10 times faster than did deaths from heart disease

CHAPTER 19

TOXINS

As previously discussed, toxin accumulation plays a critical role in the development of Alzheimer's and cognitive decline. As you have learned, it is one of the six main causative classifications of Alzheimer's.

We live in a toxic world. While you may think that such toxins can be handled by the body (your body is incredibly resilient) we now accumulate more toxins over our lifetime than ever before. Again, think of the health continuum where the effects of these toxins build up long before you ever experience any symptoms. This explains one of the critical mistakes some "experts" make where they claim a substance is safe in small quantities yet fail to appreciate its accumulation combined with other toxins over a lifetime. These same experts (and governments) also fail to appreciate that some people are more sensitive than others.

Whether through mercury and aluminum from exposure to dental fillings, vaccines and even the consumption of fish, the fluoridation of our water, pollution in the atmosphere or bio-toxins from mold and Lyme disease, our brains have accumulated a lifetime of toxins. Finally, remember that these toxins store in fat and your brain is mainly comprised of fat. As such, next time your friend says "oh, come on, a little won't kill you", the truth is that over the course of your life it may, in fact, kill you.

Since we're unlikely to choose to spend our lives living in a plastic bubble to avoid our environment, we need to avoid as many of the following as possible combined with the detoxification process that will be described in chapter 29.

Sugar – We now know that it was back in the 1960s that scientists at Harvard University were actually paid to falsify data about the adverse health effects of simple sugar consumption and instead point the finger at the consumption of fat. Today, the science is clear. While healthy fats are an essential component of a healthy diet, sugar consumption in the excess amounts society consumes today leads to insulin resistance, diabetes, glycation and so many other adverse effects on our health.

Artificial sweeteners – While the FDA has approved the use of five artificial sweeteners (aspartame, sucralose, saccharin, neotame and acesulfame) with approval from the American Heart Association and the American Diabetes Association, they are in fact terrible for your health and will increase your risk of Alzheimer's disease. The FDA receives more complaints (10,000) about the side-effects of Aspartame than about any other substance.

Food choices – Even when we believe we're making healthy food choices, we can unknowingly be contributing to the progression of Alzheimer's. As healthy as we believe fish to be, the high level of mercury found in many types is actually hazardous to our health. White albacore tuna should be eaten less than once a week and king mackerel, swordfish, orange roughy, marlin, shark and tilefish should be avoided. For a detailed list of acceptable fish consumption visit nrdc.org.

Heavy metals and biotoxins – whether exposure to aluminum, mercury and other metals, the mold and asbestos unknowingly present in your house or contracting Lyme disease, these are all toxic to your brain and your health. Genetics may play a key role here as 22% of the population has a genetic variant that increases their susceptibility to bio-toxins. This may explain why two people can sleep in the same house containing mold where one experiences significant symptoms and the other does not.

Air pollution and water pollution – Using the appropriate filters in your home and even choosing where you live can make a significant change in toxin exposure.

Pesticides, preservatives, chemicals and GMOs – Choose organic and local wherever possible. Avoid processed foods. Investigate where and how your foods are prepared. Read your food labels or better yet, choose foods that don't really require a food label, i.e. an avocado.

Cosmetics and cleaning products - the purpose of this book is not to provide an extensive list but it is finally becoming common knowledge that many people are literally putting poison on their bodies in the name of beauty. Choose natural products (read the label carefully) or go natural.

Stress – Toxins are not just physical substances but can also be emotional in nature that cause physical changes in your body and brain (see chapter 32). This gives another meaning to the phrase "living in a toxic environment". Ensure that you manage your stress wisely and have multiple ways in which to do this such as exercise, meditation, music and more. A satisfying social network is of key importance with good friends and family relationships.

Cell Phones – the research is becoming more and more clear where exposure to the ever increasing use of cell phones and radio frequencies is having adverse effects on brain function. If you're not a believer, you should know that cell phone use has been classified as a class 2B carcinogen (a possible human carcinogen) by the International Agency for Research on Cancer (IARC) since 2011. More recently, as of July 2017, Dr. Anthony B. Miller, an expert cancer researcher and advisor to the World Health Organization International Agency for Research on Cancer (WHO/IARC), has issued his scientific opinion that radiofrequency radiation from any source – such as the signals emitted by cell phones, other wireless and cordless and sensor devices, and wireless networks – fully meets criteria to be classified as a Group 1 carcinogen to humans. "The evidence indicating wireless is carcinogenic has increased and can no longer be ignored."

Drugs – as discussed in detail in chapter 8, both prescription and over-the-counter drugs can be toxic to the body and the brain actually contributing to Alzheimer's.

Your parents – Yes, I appreciate there may be a joke here for some, but appreciate that your toxic lifestyle will affect your offspring where certain toxins can be passed on for as much as 3 to 4 generations. As such, some experts now believe that Alzheimer's prevention should begin in the womb.

To help counteract some of these toxins, there is specific daily vitamin supplementation one should take to help enhance the body's detoxification processes as well as the process that I will discuss shortly.

Health Fact #7:

Alzheimer's has an annual cost of $277 Billion. It is estimated to exceed $1 Trillion by the year 2050.

CHAPTER 20
TRAUMA

As you will read later in this chapter, even the National Football League denied the role of head trauma and concussion as a causative factor in Alzheimer's and other forms of dementia. We of course know this to be a ludicrous belief and obviously motivated by money. It only stands to reason that if you damage something it will wear and tear faster. Whether it's repeated helmet contact in sports such as football and hockey, equestrian and biking falls, head blows in boxing and martial arts, headers in soccer or a multitude of falls and accidents, damage to the brain will occur with either single or repeated blows causing both inflammation and excess wear and tear.

Mike Webster's Story (Pittsburgh Steelers)

Whereas the National Football League denied it for years and others are still waiting for more "proof", if you've read to this point in the book the answer is obvious. You know beyond a shadow of a doubt that head trauma including concussion, whiplash, falls, blows to the head and other sports injuries, play a role in Alzheimer's and dementia.

In the movie <u>Concussion</u>, Will Smith played pathologist Dr. Bennet Omalu who was the first to prove that blows to the head - especially repeated blows - play a role in degenerative brain disease. This only makes sense. Given what you now know about the brain, if its structure is damaged, it cannot possibly function properly.

The first NFL player that Dr. Omalu autopsied in real life was Pittsburgh Steeler legend Mike Webster. Mike Webster, a member of the Pro Football Hall of Fame, won four Super Bowl rings and is considered by many to be the best center of all time. While he initially shrugged off his many blows to the head (playing center this would happen on almost every play), the repeated trauma eventually caught up to him until his death at age 50.

Reader's Digest wrote about Webster's life in its March 2003 issue. It is estimated that he suffered thousands of blows to the head over his career. According to the article, while revered as a Pittsburgh hero and icon, Webster kept notes of his mental state as "...deep, confusing, twisting fishing line tangled up mess of confusing things go on all the time."

"The years of being butted repeatedly on the head took a brutal toll. An avid reader, Webster could still devour books on Winston Churchill and World War II, yet his memory was so fragmented he couldn't remember the simplest things, sometimes sleeping in his car by the side of the road because he didn't know how to get home."

Webster was known as "Iron Mike" where he was expected to be the tough guy. He showed up to one game on crutches with torn cartilage in his knee, still played, and had surgery after the game. "But play after play, year after year, Webster slammed into much bigger players, their helmets crashing into his like battering rams, their forearms pounding his head. And the beating left its own legacy. "He got his bell rung all the time, just like the rest of us," says former teammate Rocky Bleier."

"After his last season in 1990, Webster moved, at his wife's urging, back to her hometown. That's when, as Pamela says, "Mike changed." He seemed physically disoriented and started to behave strangely. Webster had always handled their financial affairs, so his wife was startled to discover that he wasn't opening mail, or paying bills, or even filing taxes. This reliable family man who used to read his children Bible stories at bedtime began to get in his car and disappear for days. "I didn't realize he had a brain injury," says Pamela. "I just thought he was angry at me all the time."

"The Steelers' now-retired public-relations man Joe Gordon says, "I got a call from the manager of the Amtrak station, saying Mike is here and he slept here last night." Gordon found Webster there, poring over brochures and talking excitedly about a plan to market celebrity photos—"This could be big"—but he had no place to sleep. At the team's expense, Webster was put up for six weeks at the Pittsburgh Hilton, before decamping to a $25-a-night joint."

"His youngest child, Hillary, who was living in Wisconsin with her mother, says that in recent years, "My father called me every night." But his two sons, who lived with him at different times, saw a more tortured side. Colin remembers that his father was shaking so much from his condition that his desperate solution was to buy a police Taser gun. "He'd zap himself to calm his nerves. He'd do it 10 or 20 times to relax." "Webster was prescribed Ritalin to control his mood swings, but in 1999, shortly after his regular doctor moved away, the athlete was arrested for forging Ritalin prescriptions. He gave an emotional news conference apologizing for "any embarrassment and sadness" he'd *caused, and was sentenced to probation."*

"Mike had dementia due to head trauma, a series of blows to the head over a period of time," according to psychologist Fred Jay Krieg who examined Webster. "He couldn't concentrate, he had difficulty focusing, the conversation was rambling." Krieg adds there was no other explanation for Webster's deterioration; the repeated banging of his brain against his skull had damaged the brain's nerve cells.

NFL legend Franco Harris went to see Webster's son Garrett play football. "But Harris thinks about the risks that Mike's son will face. "A lot of guys look back, and they love the game," says Harris. "But there are some who can't walk, who find it hard to do simple things. You can't help but wonder, is it worth it?

Does one avoid all sport given this risk and all the health benefits that sport provides? That's a personal question for you to consider. What one does at the very least is to take all necessary precautions, make use of all safety equipment, ensure all rules are observed and instill the importance, awareness and consequences of head trauma.

PART FOUR

THE SIMPLE 7 STEP SOLUTION TO PREVENT THE NIGHTMARE OF ALZHEIMER'S

CHAPTER 21

THE SIMPLE 7 STEP SOLUTION TO PREVENT THE NIGHTMARE OF ALZHEIMER'S THE OVERVIEW

By now it should be crystal clear that society will never solve Alzheimer's disease by looking for yet another drug or vaccine that will remove or prevent amyloid plaques or Tau proteins because that's not what causes Alzheimer's in the first place, rather it's the body's protective mechanism. Given that, think of the billions of dollars that have been wasted and could have been put to better use but far more importantly, think of all the suffering and life-changing damage that could have been prevented.

As you now know, there are at least 36 factors that lead to Alzheimer's and as such, you cannot treat Alzheimer's the same way in every person because there are multiple causes of the pathological process. You can, however, identify your particular factors that require more focus and address all of the factors simultaneously to prevent Alzheimer's in the first place. And by the way, there is one major side effect to this program; you'll be healthier overall as addressing all of these seven steps will also move you towards optimal health as well as address many other disease processes.

Now let's be perfectly clear; while the Simple 7 Step Solution to Prevent the Nightmare of Alzheimer's is quite straightforward, for many, it will require a significant change in their efforts and habits. After all - to be blunt - if one had super healthy habits their entire lifetime, one likely wouldn't be in this position in the first place. The Simple 7 Step Solution to Prevent the Nightmare of Alzheimer's is logical and scientifically based.

Step 1 – The 3 "A"s - Awareness, Acceptance & Action

The first hurdle for many will be to simply realize that, contrary to medical dogma and the drug companies, Alzheimer's is preventable and its prevention can be accomplished without prescription drugs and without waiting for a "miracle cure". By reading this book you now have awareness of this fact. It's now up to you to accept it and more importantly take action. I appreciate that step 1 sounds simple, but without it, nothing will happen.

Step 2 - Proper Diagnosis

No, I don't mean the standard diagnosis from the standard medical community confirming that you have beta-amyloid plaques or that you failed a standard cognitive test and thus you have Alzheimer's. Your spouse and family were likely aware of this years earlier. What I do mean is the advanced testing by true experts in the Alzheimer's field and the appropriate testing specific to each of the 6 major categories and 36 factors of the true causes of Alzheimer's.

I will discuss this in greater detail in the next chapter.

Step 3 - The Healthy Brain Diet

Given the importance of nutrition for optimal brain function as well as its importance in repairing damage that has already occurred, proper nutrition is essential to prevent Alzheimer's. Brain function, brain structure, neurotransmitter synthesis, repair, toxin removal and so much more require the proper nutrients for these reactions to occur.

I will discuss this in detail shortly.

Step 4 - Specific Vitamin Supplementation Protocols

As you will read in the upcoming chapters, specific targeted quality vitamin supplementation is necessary in addition to proper diet to maintain the healthy functioning of proper brain activity as well as preventing degeneration. This is not opinion but rather scientific fact of physiological processes that occur along specific chemical pathways. I will also guide you on how to choose your vitamin suppliers wisely.

Step 5 - Detoxifying the Brain

You are now aware that we live in a toxic world with hundreds of thousands of chemicals and pesticides that we are exposed to on a daily basis. These are, without a doubt, hazardous to our health and well-being and will affect different people at different rates with some being far more sensitive than others. Toxins love to bind in fat and our brain is comprised of a large percentage of fat.

These toxins must not only be avoided, they must be removed from our brain utilizing very specific detoxification protocols that go well beyond any standard detox program. This will be discussed in detail.

Step 6 - Restoration and Optimization of the Gut Biome

Although this concept has been around for a while, it is considered fairly new or unknown to most doctors (maybe we'll see its acceptance in 17 years). You have more bacteria in your body than you do cells and the health of these bacteria play a major role in both brain health and your overall health both directly and indirectly. This will be explained in greater detail.

Step 7 - Follow all of the other five of the Keys to Health

By now you should realize that true health requires a multi-faceted approach. Sleep, nutrition, exercise, nervous system function, your thoughts and how you handle stress on a daily basis will have an impact on brain function on a daily basis. As such, each of the keys to health must be practiced to optimize brain function and prevent Alzheimer's. This will be discussed in greater detail.

How long does it take?

Most people have never given much thought to their brain health and few have taken any concrete action involving all of the necessary steps. To the contrary, they have spent many years unknowingly slowly progressing towards Alzheimer's. As such, there is no quick cure that many are hoping will happen one day. This is one reason that many are still looking for the magical drug cure – it would be quick and require very little effort on their part. If your goal is to prevent Alzheimer's, start today. If you already have symptoms, expect a minimum of 6 to 12 months of following all seven steps to begin seeing improvement.

Health Fact #8:

1 in 3 seniors dies with Alzheimer's or some other form of dementia.

CHAPTER 22
PROPER DIAGNOSIS

As previously discussed, continuing to do the wrong testing will never prevent Alzheimer's and almost always brings a diagnosis far too late.

Well-known cognitive tests including the MOCA and MMSE as well as "advanced" testing including MRIs and PET scans serve little purpose as they are far too little, far too late.

Ideally, if one follows a lifetime of optimal health, a diagnosis will never be necessary. However, given that most people have not done this, your chances of prevention can be greatly improved by testing to determine if any of the six major causes of Alzheimer's currently apply to you.

The Six Major Causes:

1. **Inflammatory** – blood tests should be conducted for increased inflammatory markers. The Simple 7 Step Solution to Prevent the Nightmare of Alzheimer's should then be followed to correct the underlying cause of the inflammation

(poor diet, leaky gut, infection, oral hygiene, etc. or a combination thereof) rather than just taking drugs to reduce the inflammation.

2. **Atrophic amnestic** – Vitamin and hormone testing should be conducted to determine any deficiency of adequate trophic support (vitamins, minerals, hormones, BDNF). Special attention must focus on the elderly due to poor absorption of the necessary vitamins as a result of decreased stomach acid. The Simple 7 Step Solution to Prevent the Nightmare of Alzheimer's should then be followed to correct the underlying deficiencies.

3. **Toxic** – Specific toxin testing should be conducted especially based on your specific history. Do you have mercury fillings? Were you exposed to mold? Once your risk of toxicity has been established you can then follow The Simple 7 Step Solution to Prevent the Nightmare of Alzheimer's to mitigate these toxins.

4. **Glycotoxic** – Are you diabetic or pre-diabetic? Have your glucose levels and A1C levels tested to determine if you are at greater risk. Then follow The Simple 7 Step Solution to Prevent the Nightmare of Alzheimer's.

5. **Trauma** – If you have suffered previous head trauma ensure that you are consuming adequate nutrients to repair the damage. Consider any testing necessary to confirm any

damage or diagnosis of concussion.

6. **Vascular** – If you have concerns based on your individual history, consider the appropriate tests to measure artery integrity and adequate blood flow to the brain.

In addition, consider advanced testing by true experts in the Alzheimer's field consisting of;

a) Brain scans that actually test for brain volume
b) Genetic testing to determine if you are at greater risk
c) Quality cognitive tests
d) Specific lab tests not typically done by most medical doctors or hospitals that are specific to toxin levels and gut health.

By determining which factors you are most susceptible to and actually taking action to minimize their progression and effects, you can vastly increase your chances of preventing Alzheimer's from ever occurring in the first place.

CHAPTER 23

APPLE JUICE AND STEWED MOSQUITOES

What I will repeat here is one of my favourite chapters from both *Nutrition Insanity* and *The Science of Vitamins Meets Optimum Health and Common Sense*.

Everything in your body is made from the nutrients that you have put into it. The energy your body produces is made from the nutrients you put into it. This knowledge gives you incredible power on how you can affect the workings of your body and its energy production.

Here's a silly example that illustrates the point. Imagine that you were a machine that was only capable of doing two functions. Your body was only capable of either producing apple juice or stewing mosquitoes. Obviously if all you consumed were apples your machine would produce nothing but apple juice. On the other hand, if all you ate were mosquitoes your machine would only be capable of stewing those same mosquitoes.

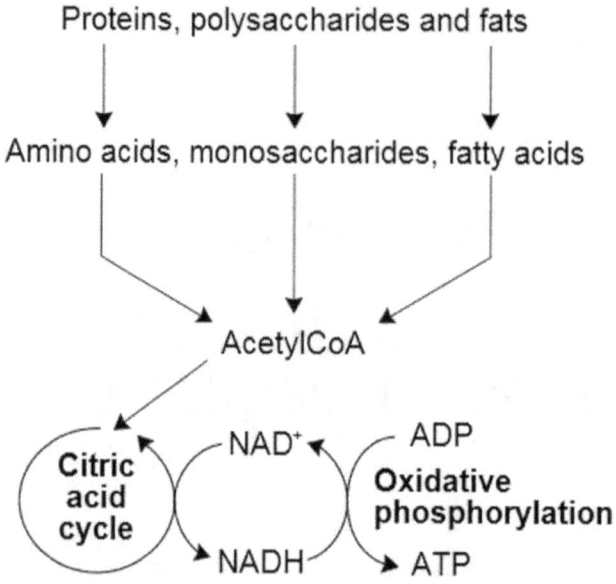

Understanding and appreciating this gives us incredible power over what happens in our body. Here's how. As stated before, since everything in our body is made up from the nutrients that we consume, we have the ability to modify or influence events in our body. For instance, the hormones made in our body are made from these same nutrients. Some hormones produce good reactions in our bodies and other hormones produce bad reactions. If we ate nothing but the nutrients that produced good hormones we would obviously influence our body to produce nothing but good hormones. On the other hand, if we continually consumed the nutrients that produced bad hormones (for lack of a better term) we would obviously produce more hormones that had adverse reactions in our body. One such hormone is a group known as prostaglandins, which among other things, are responsible for inflammation in our body. If we consume foods that are utilized by the body to produce chemicals that result in more inflammation, then obviously we would increase the inflammatory response in our body. On the other hand, if we minimized the constituents necessary to produce an inflammatory reaction, we would have less inflammation occur in our body. If we could accomplish this there would be no need for anti-inflammatory drugs and the seriously adverse reactions that accompany them. This can also be said of many other reactions that occur in the body.

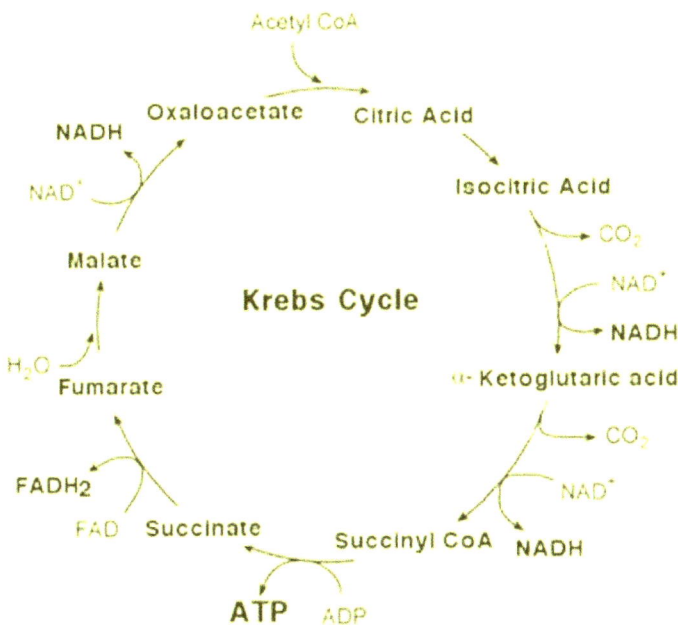

The same is also said for energy production by all cells. Without getting into the specifics of the Kreb's Cycle, nutrients produce one compound that is transformed into another compound and so on and so on, all with the requirement of specific substances (cofactors)

along the way. Manipulating these in our favour (eating more good food and taking vitamin supplementation while eating less bad food) can have profound positive effects on our body and our brain.

It's time to eat more apples and fewer mosquitoes

CHAPTER 24

THE HEALTHY BRAIN DIET

I'm reluctant to call this the Healthy Brain "Diet" simply because so many people have misused the word diet to think that it must be a temporary measure. On the contrary, a lifetime of optimal brain health requires a lifetime of good nutrition. A discussion just on nutrition could fill a book and has obviously filled many books to date. The key aspect to know is that proper nutrition is essential for health and certainly brain health. This has been confirmed by a multitude of scientific studies. Every cell, tissue and organ in your body is composed of the nutrients that you consume. Your body is ever-changing but can only make do with what you supply. If everyone was following good nutritional habits, McDonald's, Burger King and all the other fast food outlets would have gone bankrupt long ago.

Proper nutrition also includes daily vitamin supplementation as well as metabolic cleansing and true cellular detoxification.

Specific to Alzheimer's, proper nutrition must include a lifelong plan that addresses all of the underlying causes of disease and maintains optimal function. It must reduce inflammation, minimize abnormal insulin response, be detoxifying in nature, provide essential fats, vitamins, minerals, and fibre and provide the building blocks for growth and repair. It must also optimize hormonal levels, decrease stress and boost memory.

Ideally, an Alzheimer's Prevention diet would include the very common sense approach of foods that address the six major types of Alzheimer's.

1. **Inflammatory** – thus your diet should be anti-inflammatory.

2. **Atrophic amnestic** – thus your diet should supply nutrients that provide adequate vitamins, minerals, hormonal support and BDNF support as well as allowing for the necessary absorption due to decreased stomach acid in the elderly.

3. **Toxic** – thus your diet should supply nutrients that are not only toxin-free but also help to detoxify the body.

4. **Glycotoxic** – thus your diet should supply nutrients that help regulate normal blood sugar levels and normal insulin function as well as prevent advanced glycation end products.

5. **Trauma** – thus your diet should supply nutrients that can help heal trauma.

6. **Vascular** - thus your diet should supply nutrients that optimize normal blood flow.

Lastly, your diet should supply nutrients that optimize neuroplasticity and neurotransmitter production.

As such, an anti-Alzheimer's nutrition plan will include the following:

1. **Healthy fats** – including eggs (yes – the yolk), nuts, avocado, coconut oil (contrary to those who have no idea what they're talking about), extra virgin cold pressed organic olive oil, grass-fed butter, medium chain triglycerides and short chain triglycerides, essential fatty acids (specifically omega-3s including EPA and especially DHA).

2. **Healthy protein** – whether vegetarian or grass-fed meats, clean fish and eggs from organic sources.

3. **Healthy carbohydrates** - especially plant-based foods, green leafy vegetables, cruciferous vegetables, ideally high in fibre.

4. **Avoid -** processed oils (including all polyunsaturated vegetable oil and canola oil contrary to the heart association), all processed foods, almost all conventional dairy, most grain products, gluten, sugar and especially fructose.

You are looking to prevent inflammation, lose weight, increase energy, lower diabetes, have less glycation, and reduce aging - and hunger will be a thing of the past. You will also decrease dementia, have better focus, support neuroplasticity and neurogenesis, which of course will help prevent Alzheimer's. For most, this will be a nutrition plan that cycles you in and out of mild ketosis where the body preferentially burns fat for fuel instead of sugar.

CHAPTER 25

FASTING AND BRAIN HEALTH

Just as important as knowing what and when to eat is also knowing when not to eat and why this benefits the prevention of Alzheimer's not to mention a myriad of other health benefits.

Just as cellular detox and gut biome are involved in brain health (discussed in the following chapters) so is the nutritional technique of fasting, both intermittent and longer term.

Research demonstrates that fasting can reduce the effects of aging on the brain, improve brain function and have a significant anti-inflammatory effect on the entire body.

Research has shown six significant benefits to the brain and how these can beneficial in Alzheimer's and dementia:

1. Reduced Inflammation

Chronic inflammation is a factor in many diseases including Alzheimer's and dementia. Fasting reduces inflammation in three ways:

a) It stimulates autophagy, the removal of dead and damaged cells.
b) It forces the body to utilize ketones burned from fat for fuel after glucose stores have been utilized.
c) It improves insulin resistance.

2. Generation of Brain Cells
Fasting has been shown to increase neurogenesis in the brain - the growth and development of new brain cells and nerve tissues.

3. Increase BDNF (Brain Derived Neurotrophic Factor)
BDNF helps to generate new brain cells, protect existing brain cells, and stimulate new connections and synapses providing better communication between neurons. Intermittent fasting has been shown to boost BDNF by as much as 50% and longer-term fasting boosts it by as much as 400%. Low levels of BDNF have been linked to Alzheimer's, dementia, memory loss and other brain processing problems.

4. Burning Fat for Fuel Instead Of Sugar
This improves both insulin resistance and produces fewer free radicals, thus less inflammation. Free radicals cause oxidative stress to the body and play a role in many chronic diseases including neurodegenerative disease.

5. Increased Production of Human Growth Hormone
Human Growth hormone (HGH) provides anti-aging and longevity benefits including improved cognition, neuroprotection

and increased neurogenesis. Fasting has been shown to increase HGH levels by as much as 50 – 100%.

6. Increased Mitochondrial Biogenesis

Fasting has been shown to create new mitochondria, the powerhouse of the cell.

Intermittent Fasting vs. Longer-Term Fasting

Intermittent fasting challenges the idea of three regular meals and two snacks throughout the day and replaces it with all eating done within an approximate 8-hour window (for instance lunch at 11:00am and dinner at 6:00 or 7:00pm) followed by 16 hours of no eating. Obviously there is some room for play here.

Longer-term fasting should ideally aim for four days without food and only the consumption of water. Obviously this should be considered carefully depending on your particular circumstances and medical supervision may be warranted. I personally do such a fast every two to three months. Significant benefits can be achieved by a "resetting" of the immune system by getting to the 96-hour mark versus a one, two or three day fast.

CHAPTER 26

DO I REALLY NEED TO TAKE VITAMINS? THE QUESTION ANSWERED ONCE AND FOR ALL

It should be easy. Either you need vitamins or you don't. Yet while billions of dollars are spent on vitamins and nutritional supplements every year, some people firmly believe that they can get everything from their diet and even others believe that vitamins are nothing but "expensive urine". These are, of course, all beliefs.

But what if I told you that I could answer the question, once and for all? Not simply my opinion, but on a rational, logical flow chart approach to answering the question.

Do I need vitamins?

To answer this question, we need to know what a vitamin is and what it does. Do you? Most people don't.

Vitamin – "an organic compound that can be transformed in the body into a coenzyme that is required in specific chemical reactions in the cells and tissues - thus they are essential for proper physiological function"

So the answer is simple. You do need vitamins because they are essential for physiological function. But of course it isn't that easy because when we ask the question "Do we need vitamins?" what we are really asking is "Do we need them in a pill form?" So the real question is not do I need vitamins (you do) but rather...

Do I need vitamin supplementation?

I did say that it was a logical flow chart approach, so to answer this question I must, in fact, ask and answer another question:

Can I get everything I need from a balanced diet?

This can only be answered by asking:

What do I need?

This of course brings us to a key part of the question and a discussion of recommended daily allowances or RDAs versus optimum health. Is it your belief that RDAs are sufficient for health or do you strive for optimal health and what exactly is the difference? To begin to answer this, we must ask our next question:

What is an RDA?

Believe it or not, far too many people believe that these are numbers derived at some scientific high-level meeting held by the government with your best interests at heart that will give you all the health you need. The truth is that an RDA is:

RDA - "The amount of a vitamin necessary to prevent a disease deficiency."

What does that mean? It means that the RDA for vitamin C is how much vitamin C you need so that you don't get the disease that's caused by a lack of vitamin C. What disease is that? Scurvy! The RDA for vitamin D is how much vitamin D you need so that you don't get rickets! (Rickets is a significant "softening" of the bones.) This of course begs the real question:

Is this your health goal?

While you are free to have any goal you wish, if you really want to have a "health" goal, that goal should be based on what the word "health" actually means as I have previously defined. While this may seem obvious to you, most people don't know the meaning of the word (as evidenced by our so-called "health-care system") and certainly don't live their lives congruent to its true meaning. One must also appreciate what I refer to as the "health continuum", described in detail previously in chapter 5. In a nutshell, your daily actions have the biggest influence on your health. These actions have effects, both positive and negative, and occur long before you feel them. Fortunately, you have control over these actions, thus you have incredible power over your health. Now understanding this, if your desired level of nutrition and vitamin intake (whether through diet and/or supplementation) is simply to avoid scurvy, rickets and other deficiency diseases, then meeting RDA levels would be sufficient to accomplish such a goal. Please be aware, however, that this has nothing to do with optimum health or the health continuum and is, in fact, a major contributor to why we have so many unhealthy people on this planet.

Is your health goal simply to avoid scurvy?

If your health goal is optimum health, there are thousands of scientific studies (as discussed in *The Science of Vitamins Meets Optimum Health & Common Sense*) that confirm the role of supplementation in helping you achieve this and how vitamin levels well above RDA levels are necessary.

It is interesting to note that there is the occasional study that is anti-vitamin and even more interesting to note that the anti-vitamin person will rely on the one negative study to justify their position while ignoring the 100 positive ones (to be discussed in greater detail later). Getting back to our flow chart of questions in discussing RDAs versus optimum health, one must now ask:

Can I get these (RDA or optimum health) levels from diet alone?

You would think the common sense thing to do would be to investigate this question, so that's exactly what I did. I went to Canada's Food Guide (the older one when I first did this) and took a random sampling to comprise my meals. For instance, if it said to have X servings of a food group and there were X number of pictures in the guide, I took one of each. I then calculated the actual nutrients I would get from those meals. The results;

A random selection of Canada's Food Guide for the following nutrients for the average adult:

Vitamin A, B1, B2, B3, B5, B6, B12

Vitamin C, Vitamin D, Vitamin E

Calcium, Magnesium, Iron, B12, Zinc

Which ones achieved an "optimal health level"?

Not a single vitamin obtained an optimum level as determined by a consensus of multiple scientific studies! Hence, the answer is simple.

If your goal is to achieve optimum health and optimum levels of nutrition, you must supplement.

Please remember that the word is *supplement*, which means vitamin products **in addition to** good meals.

Eating according to Canada's Food Guide does not achieve an optimal level of health for any vitamin.

But what if you're really stubborn and stuck in your old sick care paradigms? As inadequate as RDAs are, how many people actually meet RDA levels?

Youngsters' Diets Found Inadequate

> "Hold the chips and pass the broccoli!
> Only 1 % of Americans ages 2 to 19
> met all government guidelines for a healthy diet"
>
> **The Associated Press**

Of course, the next question is:

Does Canada's Food Guide meet all RDA levels?

Believe it or not, our random sampling found that following Canada's Food Guide did not even meet RDA levels for vitamins E, B5 and B12. Please note that Canada's Food Guide also did not originate at that high-level meeting with your best interests at heart. Rather, it originated during World War II as a food rationing program. While it was updated in 2007 and again in 2018, it is still woefully inadequate. Hence, while it is a nice belief that you get everything you need from your meals, it's simply not true 99.9 % of the time. There are numerous factors that affect nutrient quality such as pollution, pesticides, soil quality, food contaminants, processing and cooking methods. There are also factors that affect your vitamin requirements, such as physiological and psychological stress, infection, exercise, alcohol and poor nutrient density.

How many people fit into the above categories? Pretty much everyone.

What about those who believe that God never intended us to take vitamin supplementation or that Mother Nature provides everything we need? I could simply tell you it's an unhealthy belief, but the reason I bring it up here is that this belief was right, except it was right some 10,000 years ago. As best as can be accurately determined, it is estimated that mankind did achieve optimal levels from what we ate 10,000 years ago. So God and Mother Nature did intend us to eat healthy, we just screwed it up along the way. What about the people who think that vitamin supplementation results in "expensive urine"? They're lacking the B vitamins they need for normal brain function. That's like saying that water has no purpose since it just comes out as urine. Again, it's easier for them to believe that the vitamin-takers must be wrong and are wasting their money than it is for them to accept that they're not interested or willing to invest in their health. Poor nutrition, or more precisely a lack of optimum nutrition, is involved in every degenerative disease known to mankind. Beyond helping to prevent disease, optimal nutrition is essential for optimal health.

Once and for all, do you need vitamin supplementation? The answer is absolutely yes!

Finally, we must go one final step in realizing that not all vitamins are created equally. While this may sound very much like a cliché, you do get what you pay for. That doesn't mean that all expensive vitamins are good, it just simply means that most inexpensive ones, including some very well-known brand names, aren't. Different vitamins are made from different sources with different binders and fillers. Most well-known drug store brands have very poor absorption and dissolution. Paying less for a vitamin of which only 3-5% is absorbed by the body is not a bargain. Make the investment and buy your vitamins from health care professionals who you trust. We will discuss this more in an upcoming chapter.

Dr. Zielonka's Health Thought:

Vitamins work – the only requirement is that you actually take them

Do I need vitamins?
↓
Do I need vitamin supplementation?
↓
Can I get everything I need from a balanced diet?
↓
What do I need?
↓
RDAs or Optimal Health: what's your goal?
↓
Can I get everything I need from diet alone?
↓
Almost always, NO.
↓
Once and for all, do I need vitamin supplementation for optimal health?
↓
The answer is absolutely YES!

CHAPTER 27

BIOCHEMISTRY 101
THE ROLE OF VITAMINS IN PREVENTING ALZHEIMER'S

What I'm about to discuss is not opinion. It is the actual biochemistry, neurology and physiology that occurs in every human's brain, along precise chemical pathways. These chemical pathways don't care whether you "believe" in them, believe in vitamins, or believe whether you can do anything to influence them. They are fact. Should you, or more likely someone who believes they know better, still choose to have an opinion contrary to this fact, I strongly encourage you to read my previous book *The Science of Vitamins Meets Optimum Health and Common Sense*. For everyone who believes that diet alone is sufficient, please watch my free video series on YouTube.

From a vitamin supplementation perspective, it is important to focus on three main categories:

1. **Vitamins that help support brain cells (neurons)** keeping the cells healthy and preventing degeneration. Thus, vitamins can function for optimal health, improving performance and learning as well as disease prevention and disease or injury recovery (prevention of Alzheimer's, dementia, concussion, ADHD and more).

2. **Vitamins that support neurotransmitters** – which are the chemicals that actually send the messages sent by the brain.

3. **Vitamins that remove or reduce toxins** that lead to disease and dysfunction.

Supplementation that drives energy production

B Vitamins

Now that you understand that vitamins work as cofactors and are essential for physiological function, everyone should be consuming the B family of vitamins for brain function and more. Why? Because B vitamins are essential for numerous reactions to occur along their chemical pathways, specifically;

1. creating energy (ATP) in the Kreb's Cycle
2. synthesizing neurotransmitters
3. keeping homocysteine levels in check as high homocysteine levels can cause cerebrovasculardisease.

B vitamins are also robbed from the body when under stress and by alcohol consumption.

B1 Thiamine

Vitamin B1 is required to produce energy for the brain. Without sufficient amounts, the brain simply will not have sufficient energy to function properly or to produce the necessary neurotransmitters (especially acetylcholine) for normal brain function. Specifically, the conversion of alpha-ketoglutarate to succinyl-CoA will not occur in the Kreb's Cycle as vitamin B1 is necessary for the enzyme alpha-ketoglutarate dehydrogenase that is required for this reaction to occur. Further, a lack of alpha-ketoglutarate dehydrogenase also increases brain glutamate, which is toxic to brain cells and causes cell death.

While B vitamins are water soluble, thiamine is now also available in a fat soluble form known as benfotiamine. The advantages of this form of B1 is that it is absorbed 3-5 times faster and is 120 times more metabolically active. Since it is lipid soluble, it can also penetrate nerve membranes more efficiently.

B2 Riboflavin

Vitamin B2 is required to produce energy for the brain and its production of the necessary neurotransmitters (especially acetylcholine) for normal brain function.

B3 Niacin

Niacin is required as a cofactor in ATP production in both nerve and brain cells.

Furthermore, niacin is also required to preserve the integrity of the Tau protein in the micro-tubular structures in nerve and brain cells. Remember, it is the degradation of these micro-tubular structures that leads to neuro-fibrillary tangles of Tau protein in the final stages of Alzheimer's disease.

Epidemiological studies have shown that adequate niacin intake protects against Alzheimer's disease. The Rush Institute for Health Aging in Chicago studied 3,718 people 65 years of age and older in Chicago for more than five-and-a-half years. They found that those who got the least niacin were 70% more likely to develop Alzheimer's disease versus those who got higher amounts.

Vitamin B6

Vitamin B6 is required to produce energy for the brain and its production of the necessary neurotransmitters (especially acetylcholine) for normal brain function. It is also required to ensure ideal homocysteine levels.

Vitamin B12

Vitamin B12 deficiency is commonly seen in the elderly due to its decreased absorption. This is due to a number of factors that occur as we age, namely: decreased stomach acidity necessary for absorption, decreased intrinsic factor synthesis necessary for absorption, the common use of antacids which further decreases stomach acidity, and the use of proton pump inhibitors (omeprazole, nexium) and histamine receptor blocker drugs (Tagamet) that all decrease B12 absorption.

Folic Acid

Folic acid is also required to produce energy for the brain (ATP production) and its production of the necessary neurotransmitters (especially acetylcholine) for normal brain function. It is also required to ensure ideal homocysteine levels.

B Vitamins and Brain Shrinkage in the Aging Brain

As we age, the brain shows progressive atrophy. In other words, it shrinks. This shrinkage occurs even in cognitively healthy subjects but it is much faster in people suffering from Alzheimer's. Healthy individuals over 60 years of age who have no cognitive impairment will typically see brain shrinkage of 0.5% per year. Those who have mild cognitive impairment will typically see shrinkage at double that rate, which is 1% per year. However, those suffering from Alzheimer's will experience atrophy at five times the normal rate and can lose 2.5% of their brain volume per year. To put that in perspective if one had Alzheimer's at age 60, by age 90 they would have lost 75% of their brain volume.

Now for the good news! The Oxford Project to Investigate Memory and Aging (OPTIMA study) 2010, looked at 168 individuals over 70 years of age with mild cognitive impairment. Daily supplementation consisted of 800 mcg folic acid, 500 mcg vitamin B12 and 20 mg vitamin B6 (all are required as cofactors for ATP production). The change in the rate of whole brain atrophy (shrinkage) on MRI showed the group who supplemented slowed the rate of brain atrophy on average by 30% with some cases as high as 53%. Needless to say, a greater rate of atrophy was associated with lower cognitive test scores.

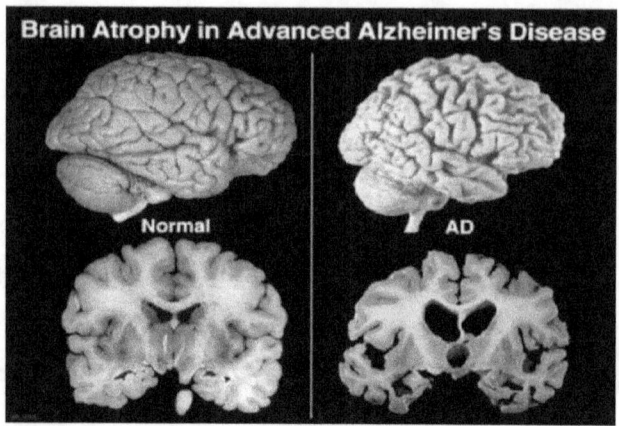

AD = Alzheimer's Disease

Thus far, the only intervention shown to slow brain shrinkage in aging people is supplementation with targeted B-vitamins. There are presently no drugs or lifestyle measures, other than B-vitamin supplementation, that have been shown to accomplish this slowing of brain atrophy.

In fact, it is estimated that as high as 10–20% of all people diagnosed with some form of dementia are in fact simply suffering from a deficiency in B vitamins.

Ilsa's Story from The New York Times

Ilsa Katz was 85 when her daughter, Vivian Atkins, first noticed that her mother was becoming increasingly confused.

"She couldn't remember names, where she'd been or what she'd done that day," Ms. Atkins recalled in an interview. "Initially, I was not too

worried. I thought it was part of normal aging. But over time, the confusion and memory problems became more severe and more frequent." Her mother couldn't remember the names of close relatives or what day it was. She thought she was going to work or needed to go downtown, which she never did. And she was often agitated.

A workup at a memory clinic resulted in a diagnosis of early Alzheimer's disease, and Ms. Katz was prescribed Aricept, which Ms. Atkins said seemed to make matters worse. But the clinic also tested Ms. Katz's blood level of vitamin B12. It was well below normal, and her doctor thought that could be contributing to her symptoms.

Weekly B12 injections were begun. "Soon afterward, she became less agitated, less confused and her memory was much better," said Ms. Atkins. "I felt I had my mother back, and she feels a lot better, too."

Now 87, Ms. Katz still lives alone in Manhattan and feels well enough to refuse outside assistance.

Still, her daughter wondered, "Why aren't B12 levels checked routinely, particularly in older people?"

It is an important question. As we age, our ability to absorb vitamin B12 from food declines, and often so does our consumption of foods rich in this vitamin. A B12 deficiency can creep up without warning and cause a host of confusing symptoms that are likely to be misdiagnosed or ascribed to aging.

Stomach acid levels decline with age. As many as 30 % of older people may lack sufficient stomach acid to absorb adequate amounts of B12 from natural sources. Therefore, regular consumption of fortified foods or supplementation with 25 to 100 micrograms of B12 daily is recommended for people over 50.

Supplementation for Neurotransmitter Synthesis

Choline

Given that one of the theories of Alzheimer's Disease is due to a lack of acetylcholine, it should come as no surprise that providing more choline to the brain is beneficial in the prevention of Alzheimer's and dementia. Choline has in fact been designated as an essential nutrient as the body's own synthesis is unable to meet the demand necessary for optimal health. While it is found in high amounts in beef liver and eggs (yes – egg yolks are good for you), most people aren't gorging themselves on beef liver nor are they taking large amounts of lecithin supplements.

Choline has numerous functions in the body:

1. Essential for acetylcholine synthesis
2. Essential for normal functioning of all cells
3. Ensures structural integrity and signaling function of cell membranes
4. Required for carnitine transport into tissues
5. Required for recycling homocysteine to methionine
6. Required for phospholipid synthesis
7. Required for lipid transport and metabolism
8. Required for kidney function

Studies show that supplementation works best when choline is supplied in the form of CDP-Choline rather than phosphatidylcholine as well as supplying phosphatidylserine, acetyl-L-carnitine and Ginkgo biloba. In fact, only two types of choline supplementation have been shown successful in Alzheimer's: 1) CDP-Choline (Cytidine 5-diphosphocholine) and 2) Alpha-GPC (Alpha-glycerophosphocholine. Another reason to avoid phosphatidylcholine supplementation is that it can worsen depression in some cases.

CDP-Choline is well tolerated with no serious side-effects even at 1,000 mg/day and no indications of toxicity.

Phosphatidylserine

Phosphatidylserine is also capable of being converted to acetylcholine and is an important component of the phospholipid layer in cells. Low levels in the brain are associated with impaired cognitive function.

Clinical studies in Italy and Scandinavia have shown positive benefits in preventing mental decline with dosages of 100 mg three times per day with rare side effects of mild GI distress.

Acetyl-L-Carnitine

The body takes the acetyl portion of acetyl-L-Carnitine and uses it in the synthesis of acetylcholine thus increasing its concentration in the brain, which is essential for normal brain and nerve function. Human studies indicate that acetyl-L-carnitine also increases cerebral blood flow and acts as an anti-oxidant to prevent free radical damage in the brain. (It also has other functions in the body.) Clinical studies have proven its efficacy in both early to moderate stage Alzheimer's disease (especially in younger subjects) as well as age-related cognitive decline.

Dosage is typically 1,000 to 2,000 mg per day with rare and mild side-effects. It is now available in Canada.

Bacopa monnieri

It is often the case that when people are new to vitamins or stuck in the sick-care system, their tendency is to stick to what they consider the well-known supplements and avoid those with strange sounding names. Don't make that mistake. Bacopa monnieri has been used in Ayruvedic medicine since the 6th century with dementia patients to improve mental performance. Its mechanism of action is both through enhanced nerve transmission and as a potent brain antioxidant.

It has been proven in dementia studies to increase the speed of visual info processing, increase learning rate, increase memory consolidation and decrease anxiety.

Typical dosage is 300 mg per day with no side-effects.

Huperzine A

Huperzine A is another substance that many have not heard of yet that has also been used for centuries in Chinese medicine. Its standardized grade is usually 95% Hupa A content.

What makes Huperzine A so interesting is its mechanism of action. It is a highly selective acetylcholinesterase enzyme inhibitor which means it works by slowing down the breakdown of acetylcholine - exactly the same thing that Alzheimer's drugs attempt to do. The only difference is that it is more selective than other Alzheimer's drugs, longer acting and has fewer side effects than Alzheimer drugs with lower dosing due to its selectivity. It also protects nerve cells against certain neurotoxins.

It has been proven effective and used on over 100,000 Alzheimer's and dementia patients in China where it outperformed Fodine and other prescription drugs.

Typical dosage in Alzheimer's patients is 100 to 200 mcg twice daily with rare side effects (3%) of dizziness or GI discomfort.

Other Memory Nutrients

Ginkgo biloba, Vinpocetine and DMAE (dimethylamino ethanol) have all shown benefits in the treatment of Alzheimer's Disease and dementia. However, they all have potential side-effects not unlike most prescription drugs that are cause for concern and require medical monitoring. As such, in keeping with our common sense approach, why take them if there are other safer alternatives?

Supplementation that mainly fights free radicals (anti- oxidants)

Vitamin E

Studies clearly demonstrate that those who take vitamin C and vitamin E at a minimum threshold dosage had a lower risk of Alzheimer's disease compared with those who did not. Of key importance are two factors:

1. Supplementation must be taken at a minimum therapeutic dose or above. As discussed in the chapter Don't Dabble in Vitamins, one of the key mistakes in studies that fail to find benefit of supplementation is that the dose was simply too small to have the desired effect. Everyone know that water is

good for trees but I wouldn't accomplish much if I tried to water an oak tree with an eye dropper. This is no different in medicine. Do you think they give you just a little bit of an antibiotic to kill off a few bad bacteria or do they give you enough to wipe out all your bacteria?

2. Vitamins work hand in hand. Hence, this is another reason why the designs of some studies are failures. In this case, vitamin C actually regenerates vitamin E and the consumption of both is necessary to accomplish the desired benefits.

The minimum therapeutic dose for vitamin E (preferably in its d-alpha tocopherol succinate form (not d-l)) is 400 IU and the minimum therapeutic dose for vitamin C is 1,000 mg.

The Alzheimer's Cooperative Study in 2009 showed that providing early stage Alzheimer's patients with 2000 IU per day of Vitamin E supplementation significantly slowed progression of the disease compared to the placebo group without any adverse side-effects. 847 Patients with Alzheimer's disease supplemented with 1,000 IU of vitamin E twice per day as follows:

- ½ of the patients received Vitamin E and an Alzheimer's drug
- ½ of the patients received only Vitamin E
- The control group received neither

The results were as follows:

- Those who took only the Alzheimer's drug on its own had a *slightly* **increased** *mortality* compared to patients receiving no treatment
- Those who took only Vitamin E reduced mortality by 23% compared to patients receiving no therapy
- Those who took both Vitamin E and the Alzheimer's drug together showed the best overall results (about 30% reduction in mortality and improved overall function)

Of key significance here are two findings: 1) the vitamin E group was vastly superior to the drug and 2) look how much more effective the drug became when taken with the supplement (from a negative finding to the best result). This is key as there are far too many doctors and patients who wrongly believe that vitamins will always "interfere" with their prescription drugs and to "be on the safe side" they'll stop taking all supplementation. Education, knowledge and monitoring each unique situation is essential to get the best result.

Melatonin

As we age, the body stops producing certain nutrients and fewer can cross the blood-brain barrier. This is true of the anti-oxidants required to protect the brain, especially given that 20% of all oxygen in the body is used by the brain. The loss of melatonin protection as we age increases the brain's susceptibility to oxidative damage.

A study published in the December 2001 Journal of Biochemistry showed that supplementation with melatonin helped to prevent Alzheimer's. Researchers concluded that "Our results clearly demonstrate the ability of melatonin to inhibit the process of forming the signature amyloid protein bundles seen in Alzheimer's disease".

In this study, melatonin inhibited the formation of amyloid beta protein, which is toxic to nerve cells and accelerates free radical damage to neurons. What is also noteworthy is the fact that people with Alzheimer's disease have been shown to have significantly lower levels of melatonin in their brain.

Vitamin D

Animal studies show that vitamin D helps the body break down and clear the beta-amyloid plaque that builds up in the Alzheimer's brain. Human observational studies suggest that low blood levels of vitamin D are associated with an increased risk of Alzheimer's disease. Vitamin D shows a variety of neuro-protective effects against Alzheimer's disease and one large major study has shown that older subjects with blood vitamin D levels below 25 nmol/L have a four-fold increase in the risk of cognitive impairment compared to those with a blood vitamin D level at or above 75 nmol/L.

Essential Fatty Acids (especially EPA and DHA)

There are many prospective studies with Omega-3 Fatty Acids (especially EPA and DHA) that have shown a decrease in the occurrence of Alzheimer's Disease.

The proposed mechanism of action involves all of the following:

1. Decreased inflammation (via PG-3)

2. Increased brain circulation (via PG-3)
3. Increased membrane fluidity and conduction
4. Decreased beta-amyloid synthesis

In layman's terms, your brain is comprised of 84% fat. As such, consuming healthy fats, especially DHA, is essential for proper brain function. Omega-3 fatty acids esterify the phospholipid component of brain cells, which results in increased fluidity and improved receptor function on the cell surface. They also produce what is known as series 3 eicosanoids that result in vasodilation, improving blood flow and decreasing the stickiness of your platelets. Lastly, they decrease inflammation and beta-amyloid synthesis. On the other hand, bad fats increase inflammation and decrease blood circulation.

THC

If you're a Canadian reading this book, you know that marijuana just became legal in Canada as it is in select states such as Colorado.

It has been touted as a cure-all for numerous health ailments, which does have some scientific basis whereas others are still concerned that its overuse will lead to a lack of motivation among our youth.

The purpose of this book is not to place any judgment; that's your choice, but rather I include it here as there is some science to validate its use in the treatment of Alzheimer's disease.

While certainly far from the complete answer, experimental evidence shows that tetrahydrocannabinol (THC) from cannabis can inhibit the breakdown of acetylcholine as well as the formation of beta-amyloid plaque in the brain. In fact, it is considerably more effective than the currently approved prescription drugs Donepezil and Tacrine.

Given the above, it must be stated that its use alone will never address the seven steps necessary for prevention or reversal of Alzheimer's.

Those who are willing to invest in their health and understand the proper use of science will see substantial benefits with vitamin supplementation.

Those who don't like to make the daily effort or make the same investment may choose to side with those who have wrongly attempted to discredit the benefit of vitamins through the misuse of science.

CHAPTER 28

WHERE DO I BUY MY VITAMIN SUPPLEMENTS?

Now that you realize the importance of and need for vitamin supplementation, you need to know that there is a world of difference in quality that goes far beyond comparing quantities. Spending 50% less on something that gives you 90% less quality is not a savings. The most comprehensive evaluation of vitamin products that has ever been done in North America found some startling results. 10 years ago, of 1,500 products, only 4 received the best rating possible - a 5-Star rating and Gold Medal Ribbon status. While it is better now, less than 1% of the vitamin products on the market are of 5-star quality. Compared to this 5-Star rating, below are some common brands:

Rating out of 5.0	
Centrum Performance	0.5
GNC Multi Ultra Mega	1.5
GNC Multi Prevention	1.0
Life Daily – one 50+	0.5
Melaleuca Vitality for Men	1.0
Melaleuca Vitality for Women	1.0
Natural Factors Super Multi Iron Free	1.5
Jamieson Super VitaVim	1.5
One a Day Active	0.5
Quest Extra Once a Day	1.0
Shaklee Advanced Formula Vita-Lea	1.0
SISU Multi-Vi-Min	1.0
Swiss Super Adult	1.5
Weil Daily Multivitamin Optimum Health	2.0

That's right – some of the best known vitamins are far from the best when it comes to quality, rating as low as one or even ½ a star out of five.

It's time to get practical. If you weren't already aware by now, you must fully appreciate just how much drug companies market to you and the sneaky, if not devious, ways in which they do so. Unfortunately, this dishonestly has had a huge impact on the health and wellness of society as a whole. But guess what? Nutritional companies also market to you, with some companies bending the truth. So whom do you trust? Please consider all of the following:

1. Choose the Right Health Care Professional

Often the best place to get your vitamin supplements is from a health care professional whom you trust. Health care professionals typically have access to supplements that you will not find in drug or nutrition stores and are produced by some of the world's top laboratories. These labs want their products distributed by professionals who know what they're talking about and have the academic expertise to do so. The problem, however, is that many health care professionals, including most medical doctors, are perceived as experts but actually have very little training in nutritional supplements. Armed with the knowledge you now have from this book, don't hesitate to ask questions. Any good health care professional will have this information readily available or will certainly get it to you in a timely manner. Ask questions such as:

- What lab produces these supplements?
- What independent rating (out of 5 stars) did the lab receive?
- What certifications does the lab possess?

2. Choose the Right Internet Site

If you can't find the right health care professional and the best supplements aren't available in stores, this leaves the internet. There are actually a handful of good sites and obviously many poor sites.

Again, ask these questions:

- Is the product produced by one of the 4 labs that received a 5-star rating?
- Is it easy to get the data on the ingredients of what the product actually contains?
- Is the site run by a reputable health care professional? What are the health care professional's qualifications? We discussed just how little training medical doctors get in nutrition and supplementation but did you know that three of the top five companies/labs are owned and/or run by chiropractors who typically have more knowledge of nutrition?
- Is there a physical location to the site? More credibility is typically given to an actual physical location that one could walk into and actually buy their supplements if they wanted to than an internet entity that could disappear overnight. My sites operate on the ground floor of the best known building complex in the heart of downtown Ottawa, our nation's capital.
- Everyone says they're the best. Can they back it up?
- Is the deal too good? It is common practice to offer a better deal if one purchases in 3s or on some automatic recurring basis and there's nothing wrong with that. However, if the discount is too high then the product was obviously very inexpensive to produce in the first place. Quality products are expensive to produce and one usually, but not always,

gets what they pay for.

- Does the site involve multi-level marketing? Guess what? There are many people who have seen significant benefits from supplements sold through some multi-level marketers and if you had to sell something there's nothing better than selling health. But be aware that since a significant amount of money goes to the various levels of marketing, the cost to make the actual product may be a factor in its quality. To be fair, a product sold in any store also usually has a significant mark-up. Just be aware that the person selling it to you obviously has a vested interest and again, can they back it up using the criteria discussed in this book?
- Is the site too heavy on testimonials? There is nothing wrong with testimonials provided that they're true and accurate. The problem occurs where there is nothing but glitz and testimonials and very little if any information on actual product data.
- Is the site selling you on fact or emotion? Unfortunately, most people, including those who are science-based contrary to their beliefs, still make most decisions based on emotion. When it comes to vitamins, try more fact and less emotion. Your health will thank you for it.

Of all the things to be sure about when it comes to quality, anything that you're going to put into your body for the sake of your health should be at the top of the list. Not all vitamins are created equally. Please invest the time to make sure you've made the right decision and choose someone you feel you can trust.

CHAPTER 29

BRAIN DETOXIFICATION AND TRUE CELLULAR DETOX

In chapter 19 I spoke of the significant role that toxins play in Alzheimer's and your overall health. Here's what you can do to truly begin the process of detoxifying your cells including your brain.

My late favourite aunt was a nutritionist extraordinaire who always used to say that if she could do only one thing to improve a person's health it would be to turn them inside out and brush them off. She was absolutely right. Proper nutrition is one of the five keys to health of which cellular detoxification is a key component.

Think of your body like a blast furnace. On a daily basis you consume a number of different foods and substances voluntarily as well as a number of other substances involuntarily. Now consider that these substances contain pesticides, pollutants, toxins, second hand smoke, chemicals, preservatives, drugs, antibiotics, carcinogens, poor quality nutrients and a number of other undesirable components. No matter how hard you try (assuming that you do) what will the inside of your blast furnace look like over time? Now consider that this same blast furnace, essentially covered in years of "crusty black soot", is still responsible for effectively absorbing the proper nutrients and excreting the toxins from your body. It is little wonder then that this malfunctioning system can lead to fatigue, headaches, lack of mental clarity, bloating, weight gain, digestive troubles, irritable bowel, muscle and joint pain and a variety of significant diseases. This dysfunction occurs whether you feel its effects or not as your body's systems are over-stressed and forced to work overtime with less than optimal results. Times have changed in this over polluted world. This is why, regardless of your beliefs, a proper detox program is essential for everyone who desires optimum health and especially so for the brain.

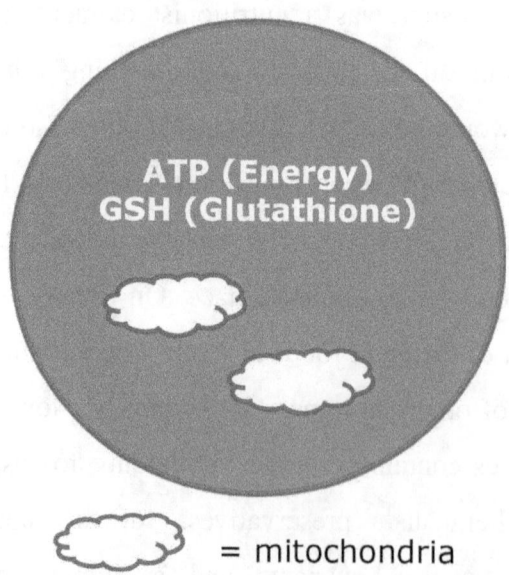

THE CELL

The exact number of cells in your body is impossible to determine, so much so that even scientists disagree widely depending on which method is used in coming to a final number but they all agree that it is in the trillions. For the sake of argument we'll go with 37 trillion.

Now appreciate that everything happens at the cellular level in each and every one of those 37 trillion cells – that's 37,000,000,000,000 cells. Each of those cells has a cell membrane (in fact two membranes – an inner and outer) made of fat that must allow passage through these membranes – we want the good stuff to pass both in and out and we definitely want the bad stuff out. Two key components in the cell are ATP, which is your source of energy and glutathione (GSH), the most powerful anti-oxidant in the body. Also found inside the cell are mitochondria which have yet another membrane. These mitochondria are considered the powerhouse of the cell as this is where ATP (your body's energy) is produced.

Given that we spend our entire lives in a world of never-ending toxins, these toxins build up over time and attach to the cell membrane eventually causing it to inflame. When the cell membrane is inflamed it loses its cellular fluidity where positive things (such as ATP) can't move out of the cell, hence less energy for everything in the body, toxins can't escape the cell, hence toxin build-up. A good way to visualize this is to think of your mitochondria as a fireplace with a chimney. While the fire produces energy, it also produces smoke. If the smoke cannot escape through the blocked chimney, the results can be disastrous.

The same applies to glutathione production where if it is unable to leave the cell the body has lost normal functioning of its best antioxidant. This is one of the reasons why supplementing with GSH can have some limited positive effects but unless you fix the cell you will never get well.

GET TESTED

It is absolutely essential that anyone with toxic cells restore their cells to normal for true health, especially the cells in the brain.

One of the main tenets of my health centre has always been that I want to maximize your recovery, not minimize your health. I want you to have everything you need and I don't want to give you anything that you don't need. As such, what on earth makes more sense than to find out just how toxic your cells are in the first place? That's right – let's test you and discover if detoxifying your cells is the real solution to your real problems.

Not surprisingly, these are not blood tests. Why not? Because as you've already discovered, blood tests are ineffective at determining cellular toxicity and proper cellular function. That's why test after test after test have all come back "normal" yet you're still not healthy. They have been doing the wrong tests on you all this time.

The three most appropriate tests that actually test for cellular toxicity on a scientific, functional basis are as follows:

Test 1 – Malondialdehyde Testing

There is a substance called malondialdehyde in your urine, which is a marker for oxidative stress and cell membrane damage due to free radical damage. The level of malondialdehyde in the urine indicates the amount of oxidized fat; therefore, the more malondialdehyde found in your urine, the greater the amount of cell membrane damage that is present.

Test 2 – Neurotoxic Symptoms

The Neurotoxic Questionnaire is a comprehensive medical history geared specifically to determining not only the level of toxins present at the cellular level but also what other health related factors can be contributing to your cellular demise. This questionnaire is a simple and effective way to not only determine a patient's neurotoxicity but it is also used as an objective measurement of a patient's progression should they begin to detoxify. The test contains a series of questions that relate to heavy metal toxicity, bio-toxic illness and general toxicity issues. It also gives greater insight to just how much toxicity may be present and what precautions to take during cellular detox.

Test 3 - The VCS Test – Visual Contrast Sensitivity

As a part of the brain's healthy functioning, it must have the ability to detect contrast between stimuli. Because vision is interpreted in the occipital lobe of the brain, poor performance in detecting contrast in faint colours may be an indication of neurotoxicity. In later stages, this neurotoxicity can cause blurred vision and other functional problems. The VCS test enables a better analysis of exactly what kinds of toxins (i.e. mold, lead, mercury, etc.) may be at the root cause of your symptoms and just how severe the problem or dysfunction has progressed. If one fails this test, it is a clear indication that the patient is adversely affected by toxin build-up and its corresponding cellular dysfunction.

If the trillions of cells in your body are unhealthy, you will never be healthy until cellular function has been restored and the toxins in those cells have been eliminated. Since toxins are a factor in most chronic diseases, then a true detoxification program must be considered for true healing.

A true detox program will utilize the 5Rs and must include brain detoxification.

- Remove the source of toxicity
- Regenerate the cell membrane
- Restore cellular energy
- Reduce cellular inflammation
- Re-establish proper methylation of the cell

A good detoxification program will open and support detox pathways in the kidneys, liver, gut and lymph and use true binders to remove toxins out of the system for good. It should consist of three phases and lasts a minimum of 90 days, most likely longer.

- Phase 1 – Prep Phase: To prepare targeted organs for the detoxification process. This strengthens cellular detoxification pathways to support toxin removal.
- Phase 2 – Body Phase: Helps to remove toxins at the cellular level and set up a concentration gradient to move toxins from deeper tissues so that toxins move from areas of higher concentration to lower concentration. This principle is a must for successful detoxification.
- Phase 3 – Brain Phase: Since toxins congregate in the brain, it is essential that these be addressed. The brain phase clears deeper bio-accumulated neurotoxins that lead to most symptoms.

Clinically, I have seen great success with such programs where brain toxicity is a major factor. If you would like to be tested please visit my website at www.DrJohnZielonka.com.

CHAPTER 30
GUT BIOME

The goal of this book is to provide a rational, common-sense, science-based approach to preventing Alzheimer's. With Alzheimer's severe and ever-growing socio-economic burden and all the well-intentioned research efforts, there is still no cure and currently approved therapies only provide symptomatic treatments for this disease at best. Obviously, modern medicine is missing the mark in this case.

Given this, one must be made aware of the growing research and wealth of new information that demonstrates the role of your gut in overall health and how this may relate to Alzheimer's and dementia. Numerous scientific studies indicate that your gut microbiome plays an essential factor for many physiological processes, including nutrition, inflammation, and protection against pathogens and thus may contribute to aging and brain disorders. What is your gut biome? It's the trillions of cells of the thousand different species of bacteria, fungi, and viruses living inside your digestive system.

Together they are referred to as your "microbiota" and their collection of genes is called your "microbiome". It is estimated that 70% of your immune system is in your gut. It is also known that "leaky gut" will lead to significant inflammation.

All Disease begins in the Gut
-Hippocrates, 300 BC

With respect to Alzheimer's, one study revealed an association of brain amyloidosis with pro-inflammatory gut bacteria in cognitively impaired patients while another suggested that the gut microbiome impacts amyloid deposition in mice.

Researchers in this field have said that "the gastro-intestinal tract is the bridge between the micro-biome and the central nervous system". While further research is clearly needed, one cannot dismiss the role of the trillions of bacteria in your gut and how the gut-biome may impact overall health including brain function and the development of Alzheimer's and dementia. In fact, it is now known that neurons (always thought of as brain cells) can actually be produced in the gut and that 80-90% of serotonin is produced in the gut.

Gut health varies tremendously from person to person and advanced testing (found at www.drjohnzielonka.com) can now analyze your gut environment specifically and provide the appropriate recommendations to optimize your gut health.

CHAPTER 31

THE 5 KEYS TO HEALTH

By now it should be clear to you that true health requires an overall approach. Decades ago I referred to this as "The 5 Keys to Health". To achieve true health one must focus on all the factors that affect it. After all, it would be a losing battle if I taught you which vitamin supplements help deal with stress yet didn't also advise you to decrease negative stress in the first place. It would be silly to discuss that there are specific supplements that can help remove toxins from the brain yet not also suggest that you limit toxin exposure in the first place. If we want the brain to heal, wouldn't it also be wise that I recommend that you get quality sleep so that your brain has a chance to heal and repair? And of course, as previously discussed, the word has always been supplementation, not replacement, so the importance of eating right is yet another essential key. All of these factors, and more, comprise what I have been teaching my patients for over a quarter century and what I refer to as "The 5 Keys to Health",

As a bonus for reading this book, please visit www.DrJohnZielonka.com or my YouTube channel to hear or watch the 5 Keys to Health.

"Humans were designed to be healthy as long as they are whole. Body, Mind and Spirit. People are characterized by self-healing properties that come from within and an innate health force. Perfect health, harmony is the normal state for all life."

~Hippocrates~

Humans were designed to be healthy as long as they are whole and they do have an innate health force. Unfortunately, the everyday stresses of life chip away at that wholeness and disturb our innate health force. Furthermore, if our beliefs aren't aligned with optimal health, we are unlikely to even realize our decline.

To achieve and maintain true optimal health and to unleash our body's incredible healing powers and energy, there are five keys to health. Regardless of your beliefs, failure to practice these five keys will have only one result: less than optimal health.

The 5 Keys to Health

1. **Proper Nutrition**
2. **Regular Exercise**
3. **Restful Adequate Sleep**

4. Optimal Nervous System Function
5. Positive Mental Thinking

1. Proper Nutrition

This has already been discussed in detail.

2. Regular Exercise

We really don't need study number 8,246 to tell us that we should exercise; we just need to do it. Please appreciate that exercise is essential not just for the body but also for the mind and spirit and especially the brain. The science on this is quite clear. Exercise, both physically and mentally, improves brain function and learning. As such, exercise should incorporate these aspects as well.

Again, it could take many books to thoroughly discuss the relevant aspects of exercise but I would like the world to know this one thought. I believe we should change the word "exercise" to the word "enjoy".

The word "exercise" should be changed to the word "enjoy"

Many of you already know this but, for all those failed exercise programs, for all those runners who hate running, for all those failed New Year's resolutions, and for all those people who find exercise a chore, imagine if you only did things you enjoy. Imagine if you weren't told you had to exercise 3 to 5 times a week for 20 to 30 minutes (as woefully inadequate as that is) but rather you were told to *enjoy* 3 to 5 times a week or more.

Specific to Alzheimer's, regular exercise will provide the following benefits;

1. Decreased insulin resistance
2. Increased ketosis which increases BDNF
3. Increased hippocampus volume
4. Improved vascular function for neuron health
5. Decreased stress
6. Improved sleep
7. Improved neurogenesis
8. Improved mood

Ideally, exercise should consist of a combination of weight training exercise and especially high intensity interval training (HIIT).

When it comes to mental exercise for the brain, many people love their crossword puzzles and Sudoku. While this is important, it is even better to try mental exercises that you are not accustomed to and that utilize multiple components of your brain function. This would include activities such as dance (learning and remembering new moves both physically and mentally combined with social interaction) as well as learning a new language. Meditation is also extremely beneficial.

3. Restful Adequate Sleep

Do you know that you'd die sooner from a lack of sleep than you would from a lack of food? Sleep is essential for healing, repair, brain function and so much more. Do you wake refreshed, energized and ready to go every morning? You should. Do you wish you could get an extra hour of sleep every night? Why not just go to bed an hour earlier? Wouldn't the benefits of that extra hour outweigh whatever else you're doing that evening?

> **You would die sooner from a lack of sleep than you would from a lack of food**

One of the key things to remember is not so much that we need more sleep, rather that we need better sleep. Sleep is also the time where autophagy occurs – the process of the body and brain removing dead cells and repairing damaged ones.

> **Dr. Zielonka's Health Thought:**
> **We don't necessarily need more sleep,**
> **we need *better* sleep**

4. Optimal Nervous System Function

During the years when you formed your initial health beliefs, it is unlikely that you were ever told of the importance of proper spinal health and optimal nervous system and brain function. But open up any anatomy or neurology book and you will discover that your nervous system is by far the most valuable system in the human body as it controls everything else. Not surprisingly, it also develops first from the point of conception. This brain-body connection is essential for optimal function and thus optimal health.

You may also not have been told that doctors of Chiropractic, while best known as back doctors, are the only health professionals that specialize in achieving and maintaining this nervous system function and brain-body connection.

> **Doctors of Chiropractic are the only health professionals that specialize in achieving and maintaining nervous system function and the brain-body connection**

How does this relate to Alzheimer's? New exciting research unknown even to most chiropractors (remember that 17-year lag) demonstrates that specific functional chiropractic adjustments (not gross spinal manipulation) actually increase hippocampal activity by 55%. That's right, brain function, specifically activity in the hippocampus, which is significantly affected by Alzheimer's, is increased by 55% following specific chiropractic adjustments as shown by Dr. Heidi Havaak in the Journal of Neuroplasticity 2018.

Furthermore, if one realizes that vertebral subluxation (the true underlying cause of dysfunction that most people unknowingly have and what is corrected by neurological science-based chiropractors) actually short circuits the brain-body connection, then correction of such subluxations by chiropractors must then improve said brain function. Lastly, these subluxations (nerve dysfunction caused by spinal misalignment from everyday stress) are usually accompanied by inflammation. As such, correction will reduce this inflammation.

5. Positive Mental Thinking

Many people often wonder what my toughest challenge is with my patients. My toughest challenge is key number five, positive mental thinking. Positive mental thinking goes well beyond thinking that the glass is half full, having happy thoughts or practicing stress reduction techniques. Key number five is about having healthy beliefs, because your beliefs and paradigms on health obviously have a major impact on your health. I'm not trying to brainwash you towards true health. I'm trying to un-brainwash what's already been done to you. I will discuss this in greater detail in the next chapter on how your thoughts affect you.

> *I'm trying to un-brainwash what has already been done to you*

The Synergy of the Five Keys to Health

The beauty of the five keys to health is that not only are they synergistic, they're also interdependent.

You could try just to exercise, but without the proper nutrients your body would never build new cells or muscle, without the proper sleep it would never repair itself, and without proper nervous system function you would never achieve peak performance or maximize growth. (That's why most elite athletes receive regular chiropractic care.)

You could try just for proper nutrition but it's your nervous system that controls all digestive organs. You could have the best bone minerals in the world but without weight-bearing exercise you'd never prevent osteoporosis.

You could sleep all the time but without proper nutrition and exercise you'd quickly join the quarter of the population who are obese.

And any good chiropractor will tell you that even with an optimal functioning spine and nervous system with lifetime wellness care, you will never achieve true health without all of the five keys to health.

Are there other important aspects of health? Of course. But most can be fit into the five keys to health. Meditation could be considered exercise for the brain and spirit or even positive mental thinking. Proper breathing is also of great importance. Are we practicing all five keys to health? On the whole, as a society mostly no. Are we capable of change? Absolutely yes.

CHAPTER 32

THOUGHTS

If we understand the definition of health, the health continuum and the five keys to health, then why isn't everybody practicing true health? Why do we not have a vibrant society where everyone wakes up full of energy on a daily basis, where life is enjoyed to the fullest and all of us live a long and healthy life?

It is estimated that the average person has 60,000 thoughts in a day. The only problem is that 59,000 of them are the same thoughts you had yesterday. If these thoughts or beliefs were unhealthy to begin with, and they're repeated over and over again, it's not surprising that we get stuck in our old, unhealthy paradigms.

How does this apply to health? The thinking mind's 60,000 thoughts in a day can be broken down as follows:

THE THINKING MIND
We have 60,000 thoughts in a day

- 40% are about the future
- 30% are about the past
- 12% are doubts
- 10% are worries about health

Of the 40% of our thoughts that are about the future, please appreciate that 99% of these never take place. Of the 30% that are about the past, we can't do anything to change them except hopefully learn from them. (Some people never learn from their mistakes, they just learn how to recognize them faster the second time around.) The 12% that are doubts are obviously neither positive nor accurate and can become self-fulfilling prophecies. Finally, what do the 10% that are worries about our health do to our health?

As such, 92% of our thoughts are not true pictures of reality. Multiply these anti-health thoughts over and over and over again and you can see why some people are stuck in their unhealthy beliefs. Realize that every thought you have contributes to either reality or illusion as there is no such thing as an idle thought. When that person cut you off while driving to work this morning, was it the split second of stress that disturbed you or was it the fact that you ran the incident over in your head a hundred times, told your friends, told your co-workers, thought of what you would say to the guy and are even thinking about looking for him on the drive home? Your internal dialogue is ongoing and continuous but are you playing dated tapes?

92% of our thoughts are not true pictures of reality

What does all of this have to do with brain health? All of these unnecessary and unhealthy beliefs add to negative stress, which has adverse physical and chemical responses. Since this negative stress is often ongoing and chronic, it results in chronic high cortisol levels, which kill the hippocampus. It affects hormonal production and robs your body of otherwise positive benefits. Imagine the health you could have if your 60,000 thoughts were congruent with the definition of health and the five keys to health. Imagine repeating healthy beliefs 60,000 times a day. Imagine acting on those thoughts each and every day. You can, because you get to choose what you believe.

These thoughts also apply to you believing Alzheimer's can be prevented or reversed as well as doctors finding a "cure'.

- If you believe there is no cure or it can't be prevented, you are unlikely to take the necessary steps to do.
- If you believe that no action is necessary until symptoms appear than you've let it progress for far too many years.
- Are you too stoic or macho to admit you're having problems? Do you try to minimize them? This just allows progression.
- Do you stubbornly try to attribute your signs and symptoms to other excuses?
- If you believe the cost or effort required is too much of a hassle then Alzheimer's will progress.
- Do you believe requirements such as avoiding gluten or taking vitamins is just a fad?
- Do you believe modern medicine always knows best and a "cure" will be found?
- Are you a health professional unwilling to admit that the

current approach is wrong and that this is a fumbled disease out of control? What did Einstein say about trying to resolve a problem with the same level of thinking that existed when the problem arose?

And here's one last thought for you. These "thoughts" don't just apply to the person suffering with Alzheimer's but also to the caretakers (often family members) who are taking care of the Alzheimer's patient. As such, some experts now believe that Alzheimer's can be thought of as a "communicable" disease but not in the way that you think. One won't "catch" Alzheimer's from another person, rather the stress the caretaker has to endure has such negative effects both physically and emotionally on them that these effects can contribute to many of the factors involved in the progression of Alzheimer's.

Experts now believe that Alzheimer's can be thought of as a "communicable" disease

PART FIVE
AFTER THE FACT

CHAPTER 33

WHAT DO YOU DO NOW?

The title of this book is how to ***prevent*** Alzheimer's in the first place. Why? Why on earth not? By now, my philosophy on health should be perfectly clear and why on earth would we let any disease progress to such a degree before we choose to do anything about it?

Having said that, you must appreciate that we have millions of people currently suffering from this dreaded disease that need our help. They have no hope with their current approach. Will my Simple 7 Step Solution to Prevent Alzheimer's actually reverse it? Yes – it can. Obviously, it is easier to prevent it in the first place and also obviously, the sooner one begins the better the chances. There are documented, published scientific studies that demonstrate that Alzheimer's can be reversed in some cases using the protocols in my Simple 7 Step Solution to Prevent the Nightmare of Alzheimer's. This requires diligence, time and strict adherence to the program.

You will fall into one of the following categories:

1. **You wish to prevent Alzheimer's** – To prevent Alzheimer's it is essential that you follow the Simple 7 Step Solution beginning **today**. Why? Because it is estimated that the multiple degenerative processes that cause Alzheimer's begin **20 years** before symptoms appear.

2. **You already have early stage Alzheimer's** – The protocols in this book have been scientifically shown to actually reverse Alzheimer's in patients as late as stage 3. However, to achieve this requires both a comprehensive approach and comprehensive testing performed by and under the direct supervision of a functional medicine or functional health doctor trained specifically in these protocols. These are not your typical so-called specialists or PET scans and they fall outside of traditional medicine. The minimum time to achieve these results (success rates are currently as high as 80-90% with strict adherence to the program) is 12 months at a cost of $10,000 to $20,000. While this seems expensive to some, it is a fraction of what a typical Alzheimer's case costs in our medical system ($341,000) let alone the pain and suffering by both the patient and their loved ones. Such programs are highly individualized, are not found in hospitals and go beyond the scope of just reading this book. For those interested in a health coaching program, please watch my masterclass.

3. **You are caring for someone suffering from late stage Alzheimer's (stages 5 to 7)** – Unfortunately as of the writing

of this book even the best functional health doctors cannot help reverse this condition at this late a stage. It is yet another reason why prevention is so important in the first place.

4. **You are waiting for the miracle cure, drug or vaccine to come along** – Unfortunately all I can say is good luck with that and please reread this book. In the past few months, front page newspaper articles, CNN and Time Magazine have all reported yet another failed drug trial. After reading this book you now understand why. You also understand there will never be a miracle drug as it can't possibly address 36 different factors. As for a vaccine, the first Alzheimer's vaccine trial ended early in 2002 when six volunteers developed life threatening brain swelling.

5. **You and/or your doctor don't believe anything can be done other than the current medical approach** – Again, good luck with that and please reread this book.

Jenny's Story

I was only 46 when I started noticing some forgetfulness but it continued to get worse. At the urging of my husband I went to see a specialist as both his parents suffered from Alzheimer's. After seven months of testing, including all the tests (EEG, EKG, MRI, blood work, spinal taps, B12 shots and psychological testing), I was diagnosed with Alzheimer's disease.

At first, I couldn't believe it, especially since our three kids are still teenagers. I had to quit work and the drugs that have been prescribed have been of little help except for a bunch of side-effects. As much as I hate this and spend hours wondering what I did to deserve this, what gets me most is that I don't want to be a burden to my family. I don't know if Alzheimer's runs in my family as both my parents died in a terrible accident when I was in my twenties.

What I also find difficult is that no one really knows what to say so they usually say nothing. We need to talk about this dreaded disease and we need to find a cure. I doubt this will happen in my lifetime but I'm hoping one will be found before my children get to my age.

CHAPTER 34

THE ONLY LOGICAL CHOICE

Knowing what you now know, it is clear that Alzheimer's is preventable in 90% of cases and in fact reversible in some based on the science.

The truth is that contained within this book is **the solution** - a logical, real, science-based solution that exists today to prevent a nightmare that you are likely to experience. And as I've pointed out, it may be 17 years before it becomes standard practice. You don't have to wait that long.

Please, for the sake of you and your family, share and take action on my Simple 7 Step Solution to Prevent the Nightmare of Alzheimer's so that it never happens in the first place. Start today. Your livelihood and that of your loved ones depends upon it.

ADDITIONAL RESOURCES FROM DR. ZIELONKA

Complimentary:

1. Please visit www.DrJohnZielonka.com to watch Dr. Zielonka's masterclass discussing his Signature Coaching Program – "The Simple 7 Step Solution to Prevent the Nightmare of Alzheimer's".

2. Please visit www.DrJohnZielonka.com to listen to Dr. Zielonka's internet radio interview discussing "The 5 Keys to Health".

3. For those wishing to learn cutting edge information on multiple aspects of health, readers are encouraged to subscribe to Dr. Zielonka's leading health podcast "The Science of Brain Health" available on iTunes and at www.DrJohnZielonka.com.

4. To learn more about true brain detoxification please visit www.DrJohnZielonka.com.

DR. JOHN ZIELONKA

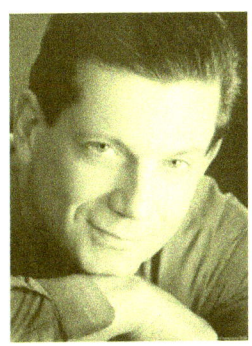

Dr. John Zielonka is one of Canada's most trusted and best known health and wellness experts. He is a functional health doctor, an orthomolecular nutritionist and is a 12-time award winning neuro-functional sports and wellness chiropractor. For over the past quarter of a century he has dedicated his life and professional career to helping thousands to not only be free of pain and suffering but also learn what true health is all about.

Dr. Zielonka is the founder of the Ottawa Wellness Centre where he is their Director of Functional Health and Cellular Healing with advanced programs in Functional Fat Loss and The Simple 7 Step Solution to Prevent the Nightmare of Alzheimer's. He is also the founder of the Ottawa Chiropractic & Natural Health Centre, "Ottawa's Premier Centre for Health and Wellness Since 1995". He holds a Bachelor of Science in Chemistry, is a member of the American Academy of Anti-Aging and is the only doctor in Ottawa to hold a Fellowship in Natural Supplementation and Anti-Aging.

He has been the Director of Health and Wellness Canada for the past 28 years and is the founder of National Health Day in Canada.

The author of seven books, he is a dynamic and engaging speaker. His Human Performance Health Series is the most comprehensive one of its kind in Canada with 69 different health topics. For the past 28 years Dr. Zielonka has presented his cutting-edge health information to tens of thousands both professionally and as part of a community service as well as having made over 100 television and radio appearances.

His patients have included everyone from the previous world's fastest man, gold medal Olympic athletes, National Champion World Cup skiers, Olympic bobsledders, NHL, NFL and CFL players to past prime ministers, army generals, judges, major corporations and even newborn babies right in the delivery room. This includes fellow health professionals from all groups: chiropractors, medical doctors, surgeons, naturopaths, dentists, massage therapists, physiotherapists, yoga instructors and more as well as having taught advanced functional rehabilitation courses to many personal trainers.

Dr. Zielonka believes in giving back to his community. Past member of the Rotary Club of Ottawa, he has supported dozens of charitable organizations and wellness groups in Ottawa. He is most passionate about his "Annual Christmas Toy Drive with a Difference" which saw its 31st year this past December and supports Brighter Futures for Children, an Ottawa-based group that helps children of single parents.

Dr. John Zielonka, soccer coach, baseball coach, football coach and adventure enthusiast, along with his wife Katherine, super-healthy daughter Breana, energy-filled twin boys Tyler and Ryan and too many pets to mention, strives to make the world a healthier place.

www.ingramcontent.com/pod-product-compliance
Lightning Source LLC
Chambersburg PA
CBHW060840170526
45158CB00001B/198